Herbal Medicine *for* Health & Well-Being

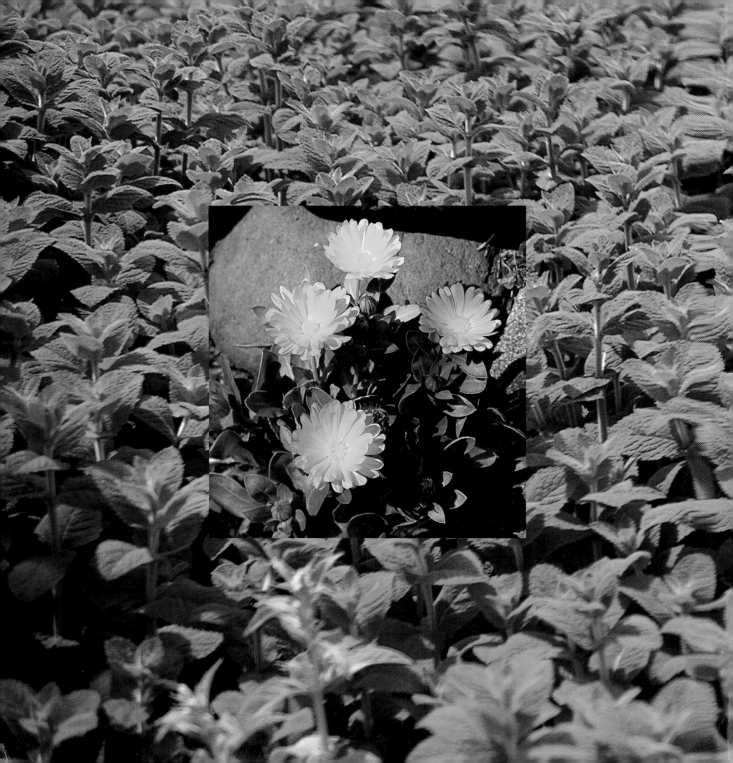

Herbal Medicine

for
Health & Well-Being

Laura Washington, N.D.

STERLING PUBLISHING CO., INC.
NEW YORK

Acquisition, editing, and packaging by Diane Asay
Book and cover design by Lubosh Cech *okodesignstudio.com*
Photography by Margaret Pennock
Illustrations by Ana Capitaine

This book is not intended to replace expert medical advice. The author and the publisher urge you to verify the appropriateness of any procedure or exercise with your qualified health care professional. The author and the publisher disclaim any liability or loss, personal or otherwise, resulting from the procedures and information in this book.

Library of Congress Cataloging-in-Publication Data

10   9   8   7   6   5   4   3   2   1

Published by Sterling Publishing Company, Inc.
387 Park Avenue South, New York, N.Y. 10016
© 2003 by Laura Washington
Distributed in Canada by Sterling Publishing

C/o Canadian Manda Group, One Atlantic Avenue, Suite 105
Toronto, Ontario, Canada M6K 3E7

Distributed in Great Britain by Chrysalis Books

64 Brewery Road, London N7 9NT, England

Distributed in Australia by Capricorn Link (Australia) Pty. Ltd.

P.O. Box 704, Windor, NSW 2756, Australia

Sterling ISBN 0-8069-1545-5

Acknowledgments

The most profound learning experiences I have had over the last 15 years (the time that I have been a dedicated practitioner of yoga and meditation) have been through my collaboration with others on creative projects. Before that, it had been my style to work on my projects alone and then share the outcome with others, but not the process. As this changed and I began to share the process of creating with others, I discovered that not only was the process a richer experience, but the final product was something much finer than I could have created on my own and, in fact, beyond anything that I would have imagined possible. Looking at the final products of these collaborations, I find I can't exactly point to the part that was "mine"—it somehow *was* just created. This book has been such a project.

Although my name is on the cover, this book is the result of the efforts and the input of several people, and specifically of one person. My deepest gratitude goes to Diane Asay, officially the project manager but really the co-creator, without whom there literally would have been no book. This book exists only because Diane truly believed that there was a book inside of me that should be shared and then devoted an enormous amount of time and energy to lovingly drawing that book out of me. This book would not be here without Diane. Thank you so very much.

I also thank Meg Pennock and Ana Capitaine, the photographer and illustrator, respectively, of this book for their enthusiasm, beautiful work, and their patience with this process. I am very grateful for the conscientious editing of Julie Nemer, who managed to retain my voice while bringing clarity to the structure and form of the book. And I thank Lubosh Cech, who in designing the book brought it all together and made the book visually appealing and accessible. I also thank my dear friend Richard Brown for the encouragement he gave me to complete the book and for taking the photograph of the author.

My gratitude, admiration, and appreciation goes to Sharleen Andrews-Miller, who first taught me how to make herbal medicines in all forms, including teas, tinctures, glycerites, succuses, powders, salves, and creams.

In addition, I thank my dear family; my parents, Jean Washington and Robert Washington; brothers, Jeff Washington and Brian Washington; and their spouses, Eleanor Eilenberg, Bettye Washington and Beth Deane for all their love and support. If it were not for the support of my family, I would not have finished Naturopathic college and could not have written this book articulating the philosophy of Naturopathic medicine through the use of herbs. I am truly grateful for the unconditional love my family has shown me as I weave my way along my very unique path, which I'm sure has seemed strange to them from time to time.

Finally, I am deeply grateful to my meditation teacher Swami Chetanananda from whom I have absorbed my understanding of wholeness. It is through Swamiji's encouragement that I have studied the healing arts, made herbal products available to the public, and written a book. My deepest gratitude.

Contents

Acknowledgments **v**
Recipe List **ix**

Chapter 1 ❦ Dynamic Balance 1

About Thriving **1**
The Gift of Herbs **4**
Natural Cycles **6**
Herbs as Food and Medicine **10**

Chapter 2 ❦ Living above the Stress 17

The Body's Response Mechanism **19**
De-Stress Teas **20**
Herbal Hydrotherapy **24**
Herbal Massage **27**
Nonherbal Therapies **28**

Chapter Three ❦ Sleeping Well 31

What Can You Do? **32**

Chapter 4 ❦ The Key to Health: Effective Digestion 41

The Body's Largest Organ System **42**
Tips to Optimize Digestion **46**
Digestive Upsets **47**
Digestion and Clear Vibrant Skin **57**
Digestion and Healthy Joints and Muscles **59**

Chapter 5 ❦ Strong Immunity 61

Immune Depressors **62**
Immune Supportive Diet **63**
Fighting Colds and Flu **65**
Hydrotherapy **72**

Chapter Six ❦ Hormonal Balance 77

Chapter Seven ❦ Emotional Balance 85

Holistic Approaches to Depression **88**
Emotional Health and Brain Function **90**

Recipe List

CHAPTER 2
Tension Release Tea™ 22
Kava-Ease Tea 23
Ten Minutes to Revitalization 24
Invigorating Bath 25

CHAPTER 3
Sleep Well Tea 35
Warming Sock Treatment 36
Neutral Chamomile Bath 38

CHAPTER 4
Soothing Comfort Tea™—A Digestive Tea 48
Constitutional Hydrotherapy Self-Treatment 49
Digestive Tonic 54
Slippery Elm Gruel 56
Slippery Elm Tea 56
Clear Skin Tea 58
Super Salad Dressing 59

CHAPTER 5
Immune Tonic Tea 65
Immune Supportive Soup 69
Echinacea Lemon Ginger Tea™—
An Immune Support Tea 70
Propolis Extract 71
Sore Throat Compress 73
Hot Foot Bath for Congestive Headaches 74

CHAPTER 6
Menstrual Relief Tea 81
Women's Balance Tea™ 82
Nutritive Vinegar for Women 82
Red Raspberry Leaf Tea 83

CHAPTER 7
Lavender Relaxing Bath 87
Liver Cleansing Tea 89
Cup of Sunshine Tea™ 92

CHAPTER 8
Lung Cleansing Tea 97
Allergy Clearing Detox Tea™ 99
Herbal Steam Inhalation for Sinuses and Lungs 101
Bath and Sweat Treatment 104
Immune-Boost Cough and Cold Tea 107

CHAPTER 9
Hawthorn Berry Glycerite 112
Sweet Heart-Ease™ Tea 113
Simple Clarity™—A Circulatory Tea 115

CHAPTER 10
New Leaf Tea™ 120
Castor Oil Pack Treatment 123

CHAPTER 11
Constitutional Home Hydrotherapy Treatment for
Infants and Children 128
Teething and Colic Tea 130
Cough and Cold Syrup for Children 132
Calming Herbal Baths 135
Warts Away! 136

CHAPTER 12
Oatmeal Bath 142
Alternating Hot and Cold Sitz Bath 143
Comfrey Poultice 147

CHAPTER 13
Nasturtium Vinegar 162
Garlic Vinegar 162
Hot Vinegar Pack 162

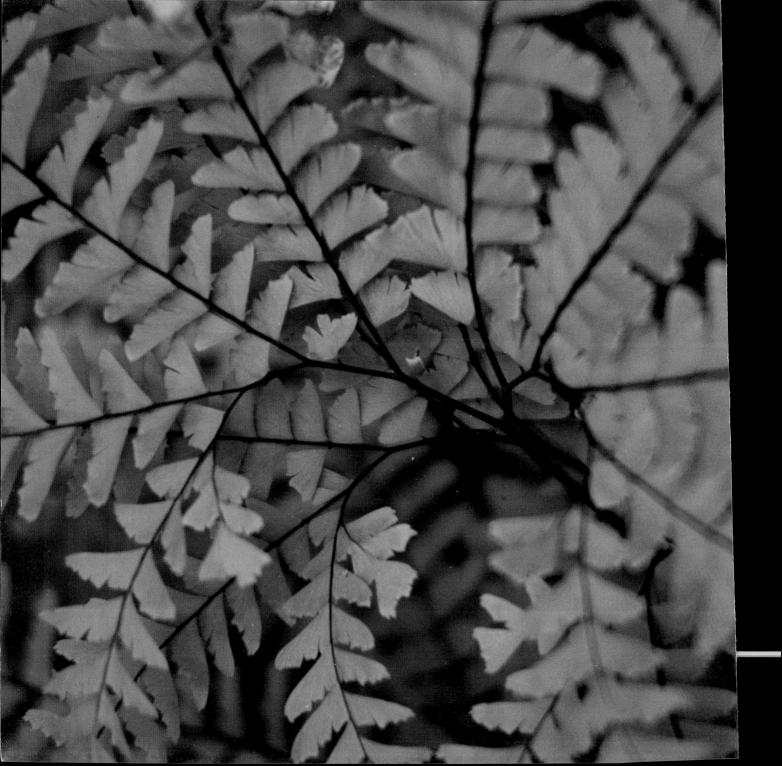

Chapter 1

Dynamic Balance

About Thriving

This book is about how we can thrive with the plants around us. Herbs are the method, but behind that method is a philosophy—a philosophy of health and well-being. Because I am a Naturopathic physician, the approach to health and healing that I share with you is that of Naturopathy. However, the basis of this philosophy long predates Naturopathic medicine. It is one that has been understood by many cultures for thousands of years, but has been set aside by western medicine for a disease-oriented, rather than health-focused, approach.

What is health? Is health the absence of disease or injury, or is there more to it than that? What about feeling well? There is more to feeling well than just the absence of disease or injury. Wellness is a state in and of itself; it is not the absence of something, but a fullness of its own. Wellness takes place in every aspect of us as living beings: physical wellness, mental and emotional wellness, and spiritual wellness. By *spiritual* I do not mean to imply anything having to do with religion; instead I am simply referring to the life force within us, which is not our body or our mind but that is us! Well-being on all levels already exists within us. The reason we do not feel totally well all the time is because of a restriction of the vital energy within us. This may be physical tension of a muscle inhibiting the flow of nutrients to the area, or it may be an idea we have about ourselves, about what we can or cannot do, that is limiting the full expression of life in us. Whatever the restriction, if we release or dissolve or otherwise remove it, energy is then free to flow through us, leading to a greater experience of health and well-being.

Health is not a static state. Nothing that is alive is static. There is constant fluctuation, constant inter-change with our environment. Health is therefore a state of dynamic balance. We are constantly taking in information from our environment, using what is nutritious to us, and eliminating what is not. We are constantly adapting to the circumstances of each moment. How then can there be one perfect diet or one perfect exercise regimen that, if followed closely and reliably, will bring perfect health? It isn't possible. Because the environment around us is constantly changing, our needs are also in constant flux and our health, the visual manifestation of that constantly shifting state, also shifts and changes.

Naturopathic medicine recognizes that the body has the innate ability to heal itself. Sometimes this is easy to see. For instance, if we cut ourselves the body will automatically set processes in motion to heal the wound. If the cut is small, the body will be able to heal the wound by itself with no outside help. If the wound is very large, however, the body may need some help. We may need to use some external support to bring the sides of the wound together so that the skin can close appropriately and perhaps apply a substance that will stimulate new cell growth.

From a scientific perspective, we can call this the homeostatic mechanism—the body's natural tendency to bring itself back into balance. We start at some balance point. We feel well. Then there is some stress to the body. The stress may be a physical assault, such as a cut or a strained muscle; it may be a chemical stress, such as too much of a food that is difficult for the body to process or a drug or pollutant that introduces a chemical substance to the body; or it may be an emotional stress, a strain in a relationship, perhaps, or financial difficulty. Any kind of assault to the body takes us off balance. If this is the first time we have been assaulted, the body is resilient and easily comes back to a place of balance. The body's sense of balance will be greater than the impact of the stress. But if the stress is a great one or the stresses come too frequently, they can over-

whelm the body's homeostatic mechanism, its self-correcting tendency, and we become ill or experience pain. In other words, we begin to exhibit symptoms.

For most people the response to these signs of imbalance (symptoms) is to try to make them go away. We want the pain or illness to go away, but may not think to correct the imbalance that caused them. Pharmaceutical medicines are designed to make the pain and other symptoms go away so that we can go back to functioning as we did before. The problem with this approach is that we have not corrected the imbalance that caused the illness. Nor have we strengthened the body so that it can meet the challenges it faces day to day without being thrown off balance and being resilient enough to snap back into balance with ease. Because we have not addressed the underlying problem, the signs and symptoms of these imbalances will return and, if not addressed, over time they will worsen, further depleting the body of the energy and ability to establish balance and maintain wellness.

What can we do about this?

- We can decrease the stresses and assaults on the body.
- We can nourish and strengthen the body's self-healing mechanism to increase its resilience.

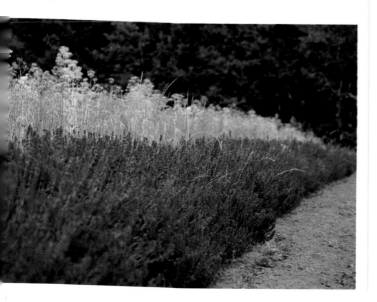

These are the least invasive approaches to restoring and maintaining health, and the ones that support future wellness. And these are the approaches used by Naturopathic medicine to promote health and wellness. The tools and methods used to accomplish this include nutrition, movement or exercise, stress management, hydrotherapy, the use of herbs, and other therapeutic tools such as homeopathy and various bodywork techniques.

This book focuses on the gift of herbs to help you remove stresses on the body and support the body's self-healing mechanism. Sometimes I combine the use of herbs with another therapeutic tool such as hydrotherapy (the use of hot and cold water) or massage; at other times I use them as a part of a healing diet as in teas or soups. As you read about the various herbal interventions recommended here, think about what combinations appeal to you and make a note or mark the page so you can find it again easily. Many approaches are offered so that you can begin to design your personal plan for wellness. I also recommend trying some of these therapies (especially the hydrotherapy techniques) when you are well. Then you will know how to do them and will have the supplies accessible so that when you are ill the techniques can be accomplished simply and with ease.

The Gift of Herbs

So many of the most nourishing plants on the planet are ones that we think of as weeds. They might not be anything special to look at so we don't plant them in our ornamental gardens. The ones that are native to our climate may grow and spread with the greatest of ease and abundance. It is these most nourishing, cleansing, and healing of plants that we put enormous energy into eradicating. We pull them up by their roots, but they still grow back. We might get serious and dig them up with a shovel to be careful to get every piece of root, but they still manage to survive. We curse at them, we call them names, we resort to poisons, and yet they insist on being in our presence. Could it be that nature has a larger perspective in mind than our perfect lawns or garden beds?

We have plants to thank for the fact that the air we breathe is well supplied with the oxygen that we depend on to sustain human life. Then there are subcategories of plants that nourish us further; we depend on fruits, vegetables, grains, and legumes for the calories and specific nutrients that fuel our cells and allow them to function optimally. Nature seems to provide all that is needed to sustain life on Earth.

It performs an amazing balancing act, providing tools and methods to compensate for every potential imbalance that is created in sustaining the whole.

Medicinal herbs seem to fill a very special role in maintaining this balance. They provide more than just nourishment to the body, they cleanse the body of poisons and toxicity, they support immunity, and when needed they act as medicines, but in a way that is balanced and generally supportive of life. Some plants, of course, are poisonous to humans and can be lethal when ingested, even in small amounts. These plants are not discussed in this book. Here I present herbs that are considered safe for internal use. There are, however, some cautions with regard to specific herbs; these are mentioned in the recipes as appropriate.

A beautiful example of the giving nature of herbs is dandelion. Dandelion serves humanity in so many ways. It is a premiere liver cleanser, and it also supports kidney function. It is a bitter herb, so it promotes good digestion of our food, and it is a strong supporter of the immune system. For something that does all that, you would think that, in this day when cancers and other immunosuppressive diseases are becoming epidemic, we would be willing to pay almost anything for such a plant. A plant that supports our most basic physiologic functioning should

be priceless. Actually, we don't have to pay anything for this most precious substance. It seems to know how valuable it is to humans, so it grows all around us. It grows in our gardens, it grows in our backyards and in our fields, and it grows up through the cracks in our sidewalks. It grows everywhere. And instead of honoring this treasure of a plant, we make every effort to get rid of it. It seems, however, that the more we try to get rid of this plant the more abundant it becomes. Isn't it interesting that the plant that we create evermore poisonous chemicals to eradicate is the very plant that will help the body cleanse itself of harmful chemicals? It is for this reason that I have chosen to open this book with a visual tribute to dandelion. To me, it represents the great gift that herbs are to human life.

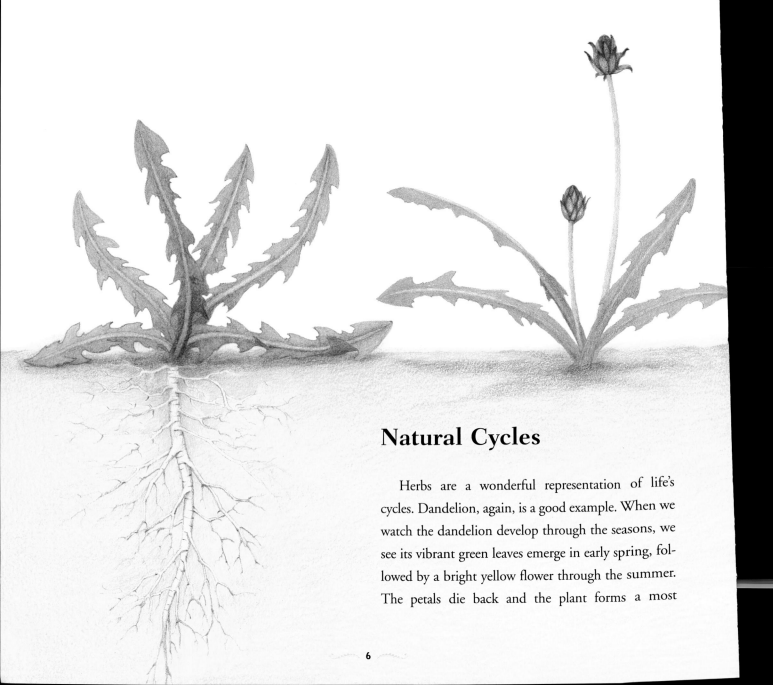

Natural Cycles

Herbs are a wonderful representation of life's cycles. Dandelion, again, is a good example. When we watch the dandelion develop through the seasons, we see its vibrant green leaves emerge in early spring, followed by a bright yellow flower through the summer. The petals die back and the plant forms a most

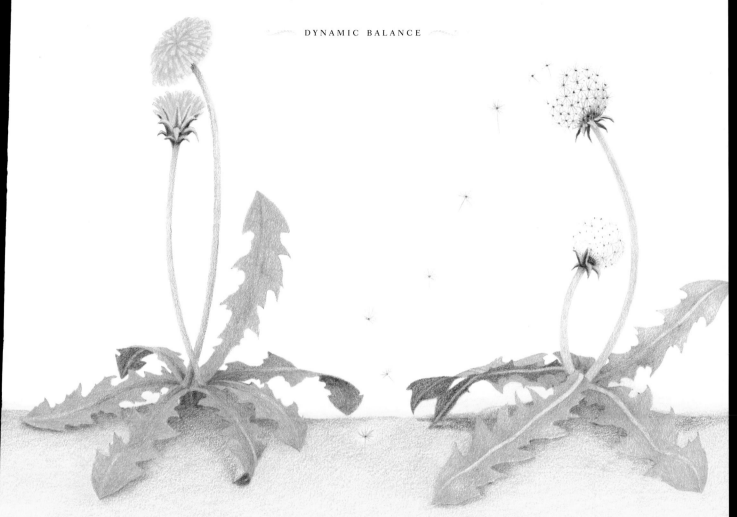

unusual seed head—the puffy globe-like form that kids of all ages can't resist blowing on. As we or the wind blows on this seed head, the dandelion seeds are spread as far as the breeze will carry them, ensuring another fresh crop of dandelions the following spring. As the leaves die back in the fall, the energy is concentrated in the roots—silent, reserved in its expres-

sion, storing up energy for the next spring. In the spring, the plant again begins its expansion phase, the phase of self-expression in the cycle of seasons.

What does the cycle of the dandelion have to do with us? We also function in cycles. We are never static, we are constantly changing. Fluctuation is ever present. There are patterns in fluctuations that manifest as cycles. Cycles in nature are easy to see. There is a cycle that we call a day that we measure by Earth's rotation around its axis or the alternation of light and dark. There is a cycle we call a month that we measure by the phases of the moon. There is a cycle of a year that we can measure by Earth's revolution around the sun or by the seasons: the expansive nature of spring, the expanded state of summer, the contracting state of fall, and the still, quiet state of winter. The seasons are expressed like any other pulsation in four phases: an expansive phase, an expanded phase, a contracting or recoiling phase, and a contracted phase. These resemble the phases of the breath: the inhale, the pause after the inhale, the exhale, and the stillness in the pause after the exhale. There is also the fluctuation of waves rushing onto the beach, reaching a still point as they turn around and gather momentum, followed by the movement back toward the ocean where they then expand and gather momentum before rushing back onto the beach again.

Why should we expect ourselves to always feel the same, for our energy levels to be constant, to do today what we did yesterday? Just like the environment around us, we have many cycles of different amplitudes going on all the time. We have diurnal variations, daily cycles in which we have energy when the sun is up and rest when it is dark. We have monthly cycles, which are clearly apparent in the female menstrual cycle. Doesn't it make sense then that we would also change as the seasons change? In fact we do, and yet somehow we expect ourselves to be able to work as long a day in January as we do in July. Scientific research related to yearly variations indicates that there are seasonal increases in blood levels of DHEA, an adrenal hormone, in the autumn and winter. The mechanism for this is not yet understood, but this finding most likely represents just the tip of the iceberg of the changes involved in this annual or seasonal cycle.

Primitive human beings were forced to live in accordance with nature's cycles. Greens were eaten with the early spring growth, fruits in the summer, and berries in the fall. Fall was also a time for digging up roots and drying meats for the winter—storing fuel for a time when it was not naturally abundant or accessible. Hunting and gathering were done in the daylight and sleeping at night when it was dark. Because the days are longer in the summer, it was a productive time for all these activities, whereas the short days of winter provided less of an opportunity to work. Winter was a time of resting, storing up energy for the activities of the summer—just as plants do. The advent of fire and then electricity has enabled human beings to control our schedules. We can make light anytime we want, so in the winter the day does not have to end by 5 PM, but can go on as late as we want. As a result, we have gravitated toward foods and other substances that stimulate our bodies to enable them to function without regard to natural rhythms. Because of the control we are able to enlist over our environment, we have over time lost touch with those natural cycles. We have artificially achieved a steady state. We can make ourselves stay awake at any hour, we can create light at any hour, and we can be energetic at any hour by taking stimulants. As we do this, we disregard the body's natural rhythms. Because the body is so good at adapting, we seem to get away with it in the short term, and, as the long-term consequences of this disregard of the body's natural cycles manifest themselves, we most often do not relate them to our choices. I address these long-term consequences in this book.

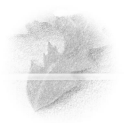

Herbs are a way for us to begin to live in tune with these cycles again. By watching the herbs grow, we can learn about the phases of the cycles around us. By consuming herbs in season, we are taking part in the natural cycle of the seasons. By mimicking the life cycle of the plants, we begin to live in tune with nature's rhythms. This allows the body to function as it was designed to and, as a consequence, with much greater efficiency and fullness. In fact, we could say that living in accordance with the seasons is the key to thriving as opposed to just existing.

There is an idea among herbalists that the plants that are indigenous to a particular region are the most therapeutic to the people of that region. This is partly because the fresher the plant is, the more potent it is, and if it is local then the time between harvest and ingestion is minimized. But the benefits of consuming indigenous plants may be due to more than just that. The local plants are growing and thriving in the same environment as the people. It is exposed to the same water, the same chemicals in the air, the same soil conditions, the same amount of sunlight and darkness, and the same cycles and rhythms. It is not much of a leap to expect that the plants that grow in response to a particular environment will have properties useful to people in that same environment. We might consider that the plants growing like weeds in our backyard would be perhaps the most therapeutic to us. Expanding on that, the next most therapeutic plants would be those herbs that we grow consciously in our gardens or porch or windowsill planter boxes. Remember that fresh plants are always the most potent. In an ideal world, we would always use what was available fresh at any given time, living in step with the seasons.

But sometimes the ideal is not possible. The best solution, in that case, is to use dried herbs. This enables us to keep herbs of all types on hand for use when the need arises. Certainly if you are ill, it is more convenient to make a cup of herbal tea from dried herbs from your cupboard than it is to go out and dig up a piece of echinacea root.

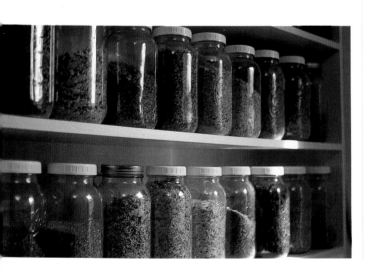

Herbs as Food and Medicine

The best form of any medicine is in its most whole and unadulterated form. That means the most perfect medicine is food. When we eat plants that are whole and unprocessed we are getting a broad spectrum of nutrients, balanced by nature to sustain bountiful life on the planet. It is unfortunate, but oh so true, that most of what we eat is not food in its whole and unprocessed state. Disease in humans seems to begin whenever we take foods and remove the parts that we don't want and add what we do want, disrupting that balance of constituents that nature created.

Another unfortunate aspect of modern eating is that we tend to eat the same foods frequently. There is not a tremendous amount of variety in the foods we eat. Plants contain many different types of constituents and each nourishes the body in different ways. Some support the integrity of cell membranes: other reduce inflammation. Some stimulate immune cells into action; others are antioxidants, protecting the body from free radicals. When we limit ourselves to a handful of different plants (you know, potatoes, tomatoes, apples, and bananas), we take in some of these valuable plant properties that nourish and heal,

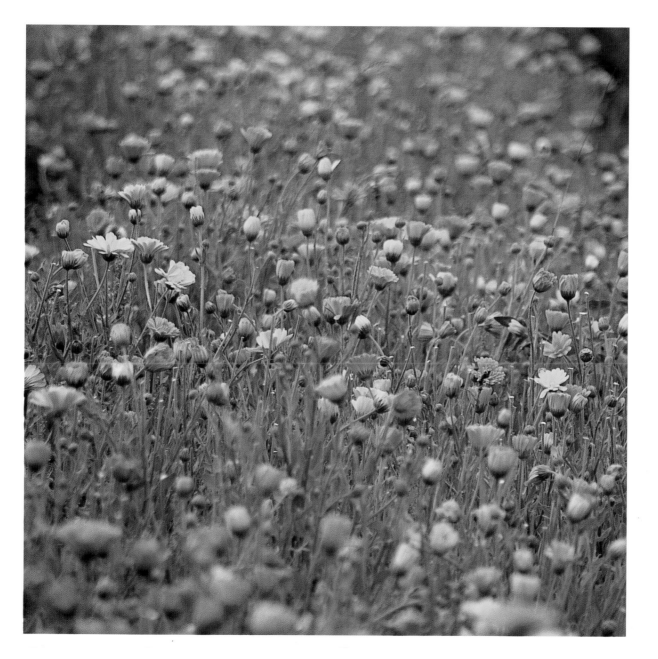

but not others. Using herbs is a simple way to consume a greater variety of plants and plant constituents. Some of the herbal foods discussed in this book are probably already familiar to you, and you may already consume them to some extent, such as onions, garlic, and cayenne pepper. In this book, I introduce some new ways to include these in your diet and ways to include herbs that you may never have considered using as a food, such as dandelion leaves, nettle leaves, burdock root, and borage flowers.

The most effective form of medicine, after food, is liquid because it comes in direct contact with the highly absorptive mucus membranes. Herbal teas combine the benefits of consuming whole plants with the advantages of a medicine in liquid form.

Drinking loose herbal teas is yet another step toward reaping the benefits that plants offer us. Most of the herbal teas that are commercially available are powdered and put in bags for ease of use. Unfortunately, once the herbs are powdered so that more of their surface area is exposed to air, they begin to lose their potency. The most potent herbal teas are made with fresh herbs just picked from your garden. The next best thing to fresh herbs are dried herbs that have not been powdered, in which you can see the flower, bud, berry, or leaf that you are brewing.

Warm beverages are one of life's simple pleasures. Herbal teas provide an opportunity to take in the nourishment of nature on a daily basis. Drinking herbal tea can be likened to eating a variety of vegetables—it provides many plant constituents vital to our health in proper balance with one another. The warmth of the tea encourages absorption of the plant's nutrients through the digestive tract; and the steam rising from the cup of tea, carrying the aromatic oils from the herbs, stimulates receptors in the nose and has an effect on brain activity. If you are taking herbs therapeutically, taking them in the form of handfuls of pills can become tiresome. With a tea, medicine taking does not have to mean standing over the sink with a glass of water and a handful of pills; it can be a nourishing, pleasant part of everyday life.

Making a pot or cup of tea can be a nourishing ritual in itself. This is the traditional and probably the ideal manner of preparing tea because it involves all of our senses in the process. Because so many of us are busy, we may need our tea drinking to be simplified if we are really going to make it a part of our daily life. Making herbal teas in a coffee percolator or any automatic coffee maker makes it easy to have a hot, nourishing cup of tea readily available. You may also wish to make a pot of tea at home in the morning, then fill a thermos with it and take it with you to work, on hikes, or wherever you go.

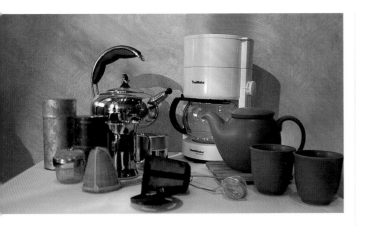

Some of you may have just recently become interested in herbs as medicine. A few herbs in particular have captured the attention of the press lately and are becoming household words. Perhaps you have heard of taking St. John's wort to treat depression, ginkgo to improve memory, or echinacea to treat colds. Your interest is peaked, but you don't know what to do with the information you have heard or how you might incorporate these herbs into your life. What you will discover as you read this book is that these and other herbs are truly wonderful foods. They nourish us in many ways. They are food for the nervous system, the immune system, the digestive organs, and the heart; they cleanse the blood; and they facilitate the removal of metabolic wastes.

These herbs are treasures. For thousands of years they were used in various cultures as food. The berries were eaten or made into jams and jellies, the roots were used in soups, and the leaves and flowers were steeped into teas. They were a part of everyday life. They provided a diet with a broad range of deeply nourishing and restorative plant constituents. Over time we have stopped consuming such a variety of plants, and the ones that we do consume become more and more processed everyday.

Taking herbs internally in teas or soups is a wonderful, simple way to introduce ourselves to plants again, the plants that nourish us in so many ways. We can help fulfill our need for vegetables of all colors by drinking teas that are made from leafy greens like dandelion or chickweed, and our need for flavinoids with red fruits like rose hips and hawthorn berries. It is medicine in a form that is not only tolerable, but pleasant, great tasting, and comforting.

Chapters 2 through 11 focus on the applications of therapeutic herbs. I have chosen to organize it, for the most part, by body systems such as the digestive system, the cardiovascular system, the endocrine system, the respiratory system, and the skin. There is an artificiality inherent in this organization, because the body, or a person, is not really a combination of separate systems working together but a single entity that functions as a unit. Every part of a person is affected by every other part. This organization provides a structure or a framework—that's all. Within each system I begin by looking at optimal function: What does the system look like when it is healthy, and how can we support this healthy state with herbs? This is followed by a look at what can disrupt this state of health and then how we can use herbs to restore health and optimal function.

In this chapter, I have discussed an approach to health that is not disease focused but focused on supporting the body's natural ability to self-heal, to recuperate, and to be whole. I have talked about health as being more than the absence of disease but as a state of total well-being—not just living, but thriving! This state is dynamic, not a steady state; it is a state that is in constant fluctuation in response to its environment. Human beings are continually adapting in response to their environment. Fluctuation is therefore a normal part of life and of all existence. It is not a problem that we need to get rid of. In fact, it is a process that we want to support. Fluctuation is the state of health. Disease manifests when fluctuation is inhibited—when our ability to respond and adapt is restricted or limited.

I feel that it is important to understand the body's response to stress before looking at the other systems of the body in detail because it impacts every system in our body. I mention this because people often seem to have a feeling of self-blame or shame when an illness is said to be "stress-related," as if they should have been able to control it but didn't. Many people have been told by a physician, "Oh, it's just stress; you need to learn to relax." As a result, they feel dismissed and not supported in making changes that will allow them to respond to stress differently. Because of this negative connotation of disease patterns that are related to stress, people are generally happy to have something else to point to as the cause of their disease: "Oh, it's not stress-related. It's a hormonal imbalance," or "It's not stress; I have a metabolic disorder," or "It's not stress; it runs in my family." What I hope to illustrate with this discussion is that the digestive disorder, the PMS, the infertility, the insomnia, the migraines, the erectile dysfunction, the anxiety, and the depression are all a result of the body's adaptive responses to stress. My goal is then to provide concrete steps or tools for increasing our response-ability, our ability to respond to stressful situations in a way that promotes wellness rather than illness. Many of these therapies may appear simplistic and you might wonder, for instance, "How will releasing muscle tension help my heart?" It is because of the amazing recuperative ability of the body that this can happen. When the cells in the body are given the nourishment that they need to function, they will do so optimally and lead to a vibrant state of wellness. This does not necessarily happen immediately. We gradually learn to take responsibility for our health and move into a lifestyle that supports wellness.

When you are in a deep disease state or far from vibrant health, you can't expect any one therapeutic approach to do the trick, although sometimes that will happen. You have to come at it from many angles. The body has to go through the process of reinventing itself, and this takes time. The longer you've been sick or moving away from wellness, the longer it will take to bring you back to that vibrant health. I don't want to pretend there are rules for this. Some say it may take one month for every year you have been sick. Others say four months for every year. But rules like these can be a limitation. The process might move faster or slower—don't judge the progress you make, just keep on uncovering the next layer that needs to be addressed. You want to use whatever keeps you moving toward wellness—herbs, hydrotherapy, exercise—the approaches that you use will evolve and change as you move toward health. To be stuck in one solution can lead to failure (or disappointment), and then you give up.

This is a book about things you can do on your own, but it is also very important to have help from friends and from healthcare practitioners who can see where you are and what might help you move forward from any particular state. This book offers you the opportunity to nourish and heal yourself with herbs. It does not replace the advice of a qualified healthcare professional. It is intended as inspiration and support in taking personal responsibility for your own health and well-being.

The wellness of the organism is such a dynamic state that we need to keep watching its process as it unfolds, reassessing at every step along the way and continually asking, "How am I relating to my environment and myself now?"

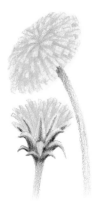

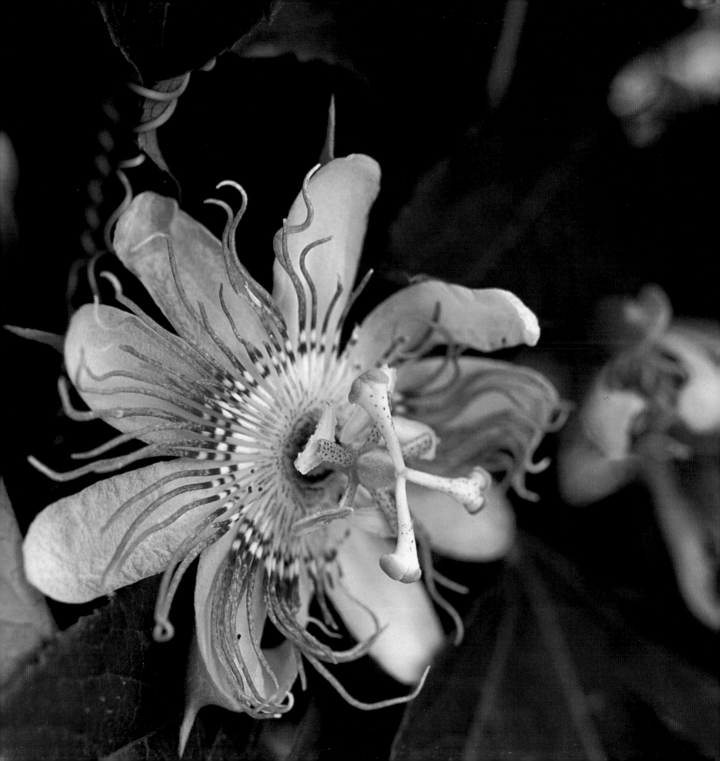

Chapter 2

Living above the Stress

Our ability to respond appropriately to stressful events is our first line of defense in maintaining optimum health. We cannot eliminate the stress in our lives or totally avoid stressful situations. It seems unfortunate sometimes, but we only have control over what we do, not what anyone else does. We certainly can't control the behavior of other drivers on the highway; we may not be able to control the number of interruptions we get when we're on a tight deadline at work. We can't control the weather. What we do have some control over is how we respond to these and other stressful situations, and we can make lifestyle choices that will better equip us to deal with life's challenging situations.

The process of finding health is not necessarily easy. Symptoms of ill health are information and time is required for us to attend to them. Paying attention can be inconvenient; it interrupts our agendas. We don't want our health to inconvenience our lifestyle. So we look for quick fixes to make the symptoms go away quickly. The irony here is that when we actually take the time to listen to the message of our bodies and respond to it, a state of vibrant health that we could not previously have even imagined becomes available to us.

When we step into health, we begin to take responsibility for our state. We create a healthy lifestyle that supports us, allows us to feel great, and gives us the ability to respond to stresses in creative and constructive ways. That place of health feels right; it is no longer an inconvenience but a choice we want to make. When we are healthy, we are able to respond appropriately to the challenges life hands us. By an appropriate response, I mean one that matches the circumstance; it is neither excessive nor lacking. Our response is not a reaction that is habitual, but one that serves us and the circumstances of the moment. To come from a place of health means that stressful situations in life do not throw us out of balance.

Some symptoms of stress are not as attention-grabbing as a heart attack, a stroke, or organ failure. Symptoms such as heartburn, ulcers, skin rashes, frequent colds, sinus congestion, post-nasal drip, tension headaches, and insomnia are all irritations we just want to get rid of so that we can get on with our lives. But these very symptoms are the early warning signs that we are not maintaining a balance in relation to the stresses in our life, and they can lead to those more attention-grabbing symptoms: heart attack, a stroke, and organ failure. I discuss in Chapter 4 that the balance in the nervous system is the most important regulatory factor in digestion. Too much sympathetic nervous system activity decreases our ability to digest food, absorb nourishment, and eliminate properly. This decreased function can lead to simple symptoms such as heartburn or constipation, symptoms we often ignore. However, heartburn can lead to an ulcer, and constipation can lead to colon cancer. The first step, the first line of defense protecting us from these serious conditions is to maintain balance in the nervous system. I call this living above the stress.

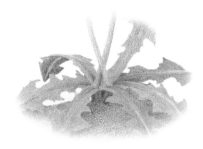

The Body's Response Mechanism

We are designed to adapt to different circumstances. You could call these varying circumstances to which we respond stressors—something that triggers a response from the body (whole person) and stimulates the body to take some sort of action. A stressor is not necessarily a bad thing; it can be just a normal part of life. For instance, you eat a particular food. From the moment you take that food into your mouth (or even before, as you smell the food or see an image of the food in an advertisement) your body begins a series of responses. Hormones are secreted in response to the taste of the food in the mouth, specific digestive enzymes are secreted depending on the type of food, and it takes more or less time to move through your digestive tract based on the chemical makeup of the particular food. The body is responding to the current situation. It has changed its state in response to input from the environment.

This and so many other responses of the body to outside input are really no different than the response of the body to events that we generally think of as stressful. The body responds to stress by producing particular hormones, shunting blood to areas that are most important at that moment and away from areas that are less important, providing the fuel and energy that are needed to deal with the situation, and so on. These are simple responses of the body to the environmental input. When the stressful situation no longer exists, the body changes its response. This is all normal. Problems or ill health arise when, due to repeated or prolonged stress, our body gets stuck in a stress response and can no longer respond to other input appropriately. To see how this leads to ill health, let's take a closer look at the body's response to stress.

Within seconds of a stressful episode the sympathetic nervous system releases the chemical messengers norepinephrine and epinephrine (commonly referred to as adrenaline).* These messengers first increase our perception and then stimulate changes in tissues and cells throughout the body so that it can respond appropriately—run away quickly or fight. At the same time, the hypothalamus releases hormones into the blood stream that also evoke responses in the heart, liver, lungs, brain, and muscles to allow them to respond to the emergency or to the perceived emergency or threat. There are many

---

*Norepinephrine and epinephrine. These hormones are secreted by the adrenal medulla; they are neurotransmitters in the central nervous system. They are potent stimulators of the sympathetic nervous system.

messengers or combinations of messengers released depending on the particular stress. Many of these messengers are involved in regulating most metabolic and healing functions of the body.

Within minutes of stress, the adrenal cortex releases cortisol into the bloodstream. Cortisol provides the body with the energy it needs to respond to the stress; it releases stored fuels, increases cardiovascular and pulmonary tone, increases perception and cognition, increases strength and reflex responses, and increases pain tolerance. In an emergency, this is all useful. The other effects of increased cortisol are a decrease in immune function, digestion, sexuality, and growth. It is also appropriate for these functions to be decreased in the short term during an emergency so that the body can focus all its attention on getting out of danger. You can see, however, that when we are exposed to prolonged stress from perceived emergencies and cortisol is high over an extended period of time, our health will be compromised. Decreased immune function not only makes us vulnerable to viruses and bacteria, but can allow the development of cancer or the evolution of HIV to AIDS. In the short term, decreased digestive function may mean that the last meal eaten has a bumpy ride through the digestive tract, perhaps manifesting as gas, bloating, intestinal cramping, or constipation.

In the long run, decreased digestive capacity leads to poor assimilation of nutrients, which can cause any number of health challenges including depression, fatigue, insomnia, anxiety, and inability to concentrate. The impact of stress on sex hormones can lead to decreased libido, infertility and other hormonal imbalances. Common conditions such as hypertension, asthma, and diabetes have similar origins from responses to prolonged and ignored states of stress.

De-Stress Teas

Because the response of the body to ongoing stress is a change in the nervous system to sympathetic dominance, our primary goal therapeutically is to restore nervous system tone and relieve some of the symptoms of the nervous system imbalance such as tense muscles and feelings of agitation or anxiety. Teas are a wonderful way to take herbs that counteract these symptoms and restore nervous system balance. In addition, the simple act of making a cup of tea allows you to take a break for a moment to nurture yourself. The warmth of the tea as you hold the cup in your hand and in your throat as you drink is soothing and helps your system pause, even if just for a moment, and take a deep breath.

Tension Release Tea™ shown on the next page can be taken daily over a period of time to restore balance to the nervous system. It has the additional benefits of cleansing of the blood by supporting the liver. This is important to help the body rid itself of hormones that are released in excess when under stress.

Kava-Ease Tea shown on page 23 can also be used to relax muscles and relieve anxiety due to stress, but it is meant to be taken during especially stressful times, not every day. It includes the herb kava kava, which relaxes muscles but, unlike many other muscle relaxants, is not a sedative. I love to use kava roots in tea. It is a very hard root, however, and needs more than a simple steeping to extract its active constituents. I mix kava with fennel seed (also an antispasmodic), licorice root, cinnamon bark, and orange peel for a tea that is perfect when the stress of the day has left me anxious, with tight muscles and perhaps a slightly upset digestive tract. It's relaxing and calms and eases muscle tension. When this happens, circulation increases to areas of the body that are tight. Increased circulation means increased nutrients to cells, restoring proper function and a feeling of ease to the body.

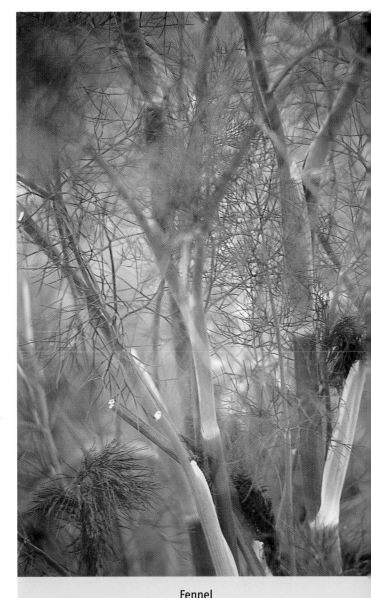

Fennel

Tension Release Tea™

INGREDIENTS

1 part* St. John's wort
1 part Skullcap
1 part Lemon verbena
1/2 part Passion flower

INSTRUCTIONS

Using your favorite tea-making tool (tea pot, French press, infusing basket, or tea ball) add a heaping teaspoon of the herb mixture to each cup of just-boiled water. Cover and let sit for approximately 5 minutes. Pour the tea into a cup, straining out the herbs (or remove the infusing basket or tea ball), inhale the tea's aroma, and sip slowly.

DOSE / TIMING / DURATION

Drink 1–4 cups per day.

BENEFITS

Relaxes muscles, soothes the nerves, and lifts the spirits. St. John's wort not only has the antidepressant effects for which it is famous, but also acts on the liver to purify the blood.

INDICATIONS

Tight muscles, tension headaches, nervous tension, nervous exhaustion, restlessness, heart palpitations, anxiety, and insomnia due to nervousness.

CAUTIONS

- St. John's wort should not be used during pregnancy.

- St. John's wort can cause photosensitivity in some individuals. If a rash or sunburn appears, discontinue use and skin symptoms will resolve.

- St. John's wort has the potential to enhance or inhibit the action of some prescription drugs. If you are taking medications, consult with a healthcare practitioner who is familiar with the use of herbal medicines before using St. John's wort on an ongoing basis.

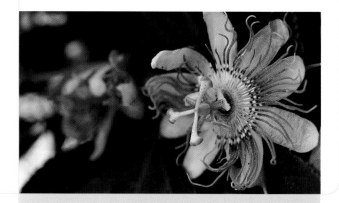

Passion flower

*In the tea recipes throughout this book, *part* refers to parts by volume.

Kava-Ease Tea

INGREDIENTS

1 part Kava kava root
1/4 part Licorice root
1/4 part Cinnamon
1/4 part Ginger
1/4 part Fennel

INSTRUCTIONS

Place pure cool water in a sauce pan and add 1 tablespoon of the herb mixture for every cup of water. Bring to a rolling boil. Allow the herbs to simmer for 10 minutes. Turn off the heat and let sit for another 5 minutes. Strain out the herbs and drink the remaining liquid.

DOSE / TIMING / DURATION

Drink 1–4 cups in any 1 day. Use intermittently, not every day and not for extended periods of time.

BENEFITS

Relieves muscle tension and spasm, soothes digestion, and eases anxiety.

INDICATIONS

Very useful for treating tension headaches, menstrual discomfort, stage fright, muscle tension, and insomnia.

CAUTIONS

- Because kava kava relaxes skeletal muscles, it should not be used before or while operating heavy machinery or in other situations in which the loss of fine motor skills could be dangerous.

- Kava should not be used during pregnancy.

Kava kava has been used safely in the South Pacific for over 2,000 years, and has been shown to be safe and effective for treating anxiety in recent studies performed at Duke University. However, there have recently been reports of kava kava leading to liver toxicity in a small number of people in Europe. This can be explained in a few ways. The European companies often use kava stem in their formulas, which is considered mildly toxic by the people who traditionally use the root on Fiji. The European formulas also extract the constituents of the herb in alcohol and acetone, which produces a much more potent, drug-like product than is produced by the traditional water extractions. Finally, in the European studies, in 18 of the 30 cases reported the patients were concurrently taking prescription or over-the-counter drugs with known or potential liver toxicity. The use of kava kava presented in this book—extracted from the roots with water for short-term use while the underlying causes of the anxiety are addressed—has little potential for liver toxicity.

10 MINUTES TO REVITALIZATION

Wet a washcloth thoroughly with steaming hot water and wring it out, wearing rubber gloves. Sprinkle the washcloth with a few drops of lavender essential oil. Sit in a comfortable chair and lay the warm washcloth over your face, allow your arms to release down by your sides and breathe in the aroma of the lavender. When the cloth no longer feels warm, you can use it to "wipe the day" off of your face.

Peppermint essential oil can be used in place of lavender. Peppermint stimulates circulation, feels tingly, and has a soothing yet stimulating scent.

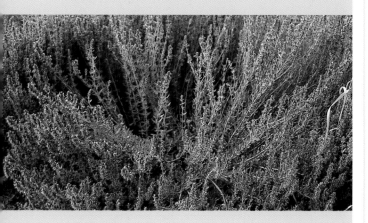

Lavender

Herbal Hydrotherapy

Herbs can also be used externally to help us combat the effects of stress on the body. Herbal baths and massage with herbal oils help us to take a deep breath by relaxing the tight muscles that inhibit respiration. The simple scent of an essential oil can bring about the same response from the opposite direction; lavender essential oil facilitates a deep breath that, in turn, helps to relax tight muscles. In a hot bath, our muscles immediately begin to relax in response to the warmth. Our physiology opens and becomes more accessible to us. We can then refocus ourselves and be present and aware of our needs as we move through the rest of the day, or we can truly rest during the night.

We often take the benefits of these kinds of treatments for granted, thinking them too simplistic to really have an effect. They *are* simple and therein lies their beauty. Some of the treatments described here provide the quick fix that we are so often looking for. But unlike an over-the-counter-medication approach, they require some attention on our part. By giving ourselves this attention, we take one more step in the direction of becoming aware of our needs and knowing what we can do to address them.

Herbal baths are a wonderful way to receive the restorative benefits of water and herbs. For calming bath, perfect before bed or during times of agitation or anxiety, see Chapter 11 and the Neutral Chamomile Bath in Chapter 3. For a bath that relaxes muscles but has a more stimulating quality, I suggest the following invigorating baths, using any of the herbs listed in Table 1, on page 26.

Invigorating Bath

INGREDIENTS

Essential oil of peppermint, rosemary, or thyme

INSTRUCTIONS

Add 5–7 drops of one of the above essential oils to a warm bath. You may want to mix the essential oil with 1 teaspoon base oil (such as almond oil) or milk to aid dispersion. Also, have a small basin of ice water by the bathtub with one drop of the same essential oil in it. Soak a washcloth in this basin as you soak in the tub.

Soak in the bath for 10 minutes. When you step out of the bath, wring out the washcloth and rub it briskly all over your body. Start at the periphery (hands and feet) and stroke briskly toward your heart with the washcloth.

DOSE / TIMING / DURATION

Use this bath any time your energy is low and needs revitalizing. As a daily treatment this bath is tonifying, which means that it supports physiologic activity that helps restore normal function.

BENEFITS AND INDICATIONS

See Table 1 on page 26.

CAUTION

- Never apply undiluted essential oils directly to the skin.

- See Table 1 cautions for individual essential oils.

Table 1

Essential Oils for Invigorating Baths

HERBS	BENEFITS	INDICATIONS	CAUTIONS
Peppermint	Refreshing, revitalizing, energizing, relieves fatigue	Mental and physical fatigue, tense muscles, muscle pain	May be irritating to some individuals, avoid during pregnancy
Rosemary	Stimulating, invigorating, pain relieving, muscle relaxing, clears the mind	Tight aching muscles, mental and physical fatigue, tension headache	Avoid during pregnancy
Thyme	Stimulating, tonifying to the nerves, antiseptic	Fatigue, depression, headaches, muscular aches and pains	May cause irritation or allergic reaction in sensitive individuals, avoid during pregnancy

Herbal Massage

Another way of decreasing tension in the body due to stress is to rub the tight muscles with an herbal oil. Tension headaches are often caused by tightness in the muscles of the neck, shoulders, and upper back. A soothing treatment for tension headaches is to rub these areas with lavender oil. The muscles are relaxed by the massage and by the lavender, which sends messages to the brain to relax as you take a deep breath. Massage increases circulation and therefore nutrition to our cells. It increases absorption of nutrients into the tissues, increases lymphatic flow and drainage, calms and soothes the nervous system, speeds relief of muscle fatigue, and decreases the thickening of scars and adhesions from wounds or surgery. Herbal oils—that is, a carrier oil infused with an herb—can be used for additional therapeutic effects. An anti-inflammatory herb such as arnica, for instance, reduces pain and muscle spasms; add a few drops of arnica oil to a tablespoon of carrier oil for this purpose.

Herbal oils are also beneficial when rubbed into the feet. There are reflex points on the feet and hands that relate to every gland, organ and part of the body. By applying pressure to these reflex points, we promote relaxation and stress release and help to promote normal functioning of the entire body. Without knowing the details of Reflexology, you can simply massage the areas of the foot that are most tender and receive great benefits.

Massaging the reflex points on the hands and feet is technically known as Reflexology, a healing art that has been used for many thousands of years in India, China, and Egypt. Reflexology is a method of activating the healing powers of the body. Blood circulates faster than it normally does and, as a result, there is a cleansing of the lymphatic system and increased oxygenation of the blood. The by-product is a more relaxed body and a general feeling of well-being.

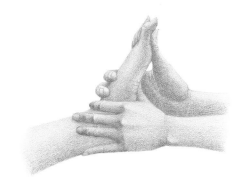

Nonherbal Therapies

BREATHING

In my discussion of relieving muscle tension, I frequently mention that these therapies help us to take a deep breath. It is my opinion that being able to breath naturally and fully is the most important aspect of our ability to respond to stress in a creative manner. When we breathe in, we are nourishing every cell in our body with much needed oxygen. Without an appropriate amount of oxygen, our cells diminish the performance of their day-to-day functions. As a result, we feel tired, sluggish, or even depressed. With optimum oxygenation, our cells thrive. When we breathe out, we are taking carbon dioxide, a poisonous waste product, out of our cells and eliminating it from the body.

A very common response to stressful situations is for the muscles involved in breathing to tighten up. As this happens, our breathing becomes shallow. Shallow breathing means decreased gas exchange— less oxygen in and less carbon dioxide out. This imbalance sets off stress signals from the cells to the brain that we need more oxygen. The body's response then is to breathe faster to try to get enough oxygen. Faster breathing requires more energy and the body fatigues more easily than normal. If instead we interrupt this cascade of events by deepening our breath and relaxing the muscles of respiration, we reestablish the balance between oxygen and carbon dioxide in the body. We feel rejuvenated instead of tired. Therefore, I believe that the most important response to stress is breathing—taking a deep breath, and being aware of our breathing. The herbal therapies already described facilitate our ability to do this.

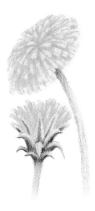

YOGA

Another extremely valuable tool in this regard is yoga. Although yoga is not the topic of this book, it is a therapy that completely supports the philosophy of wellness that is given here, and deserves a brief mention. The breathing, stretching, and strengthening that happens in yoga give us not only the ability to move with more ease, but also to consciously use our breathing to manage stressful situations and to find our center; it also gives us the ability to express ourselves clearly in every area of our lives. Expressing ourselves clearly is one of the ways we can deal with potentially stressful events so that tensions do not accumulate in our bodies. Through yoga we learn to observe ourselves and our reactions to things, and observing ourselves is the first step to being able to respond differently. Breath focus teaches us to be aware of how events affect us so that we can respond in a way that feels right to us, not in a patterned response. When we are relaxed and centered, we are in touch with our true self and more able to be guided by it.

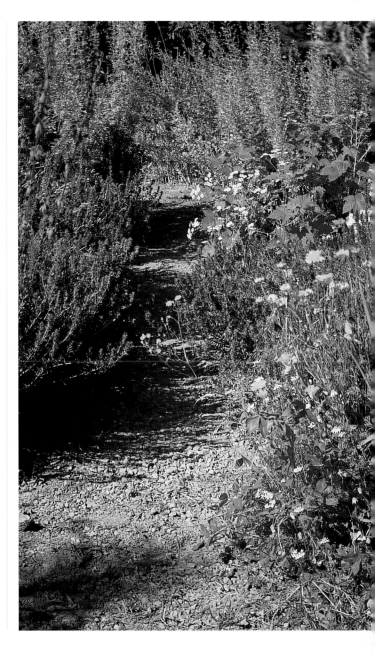

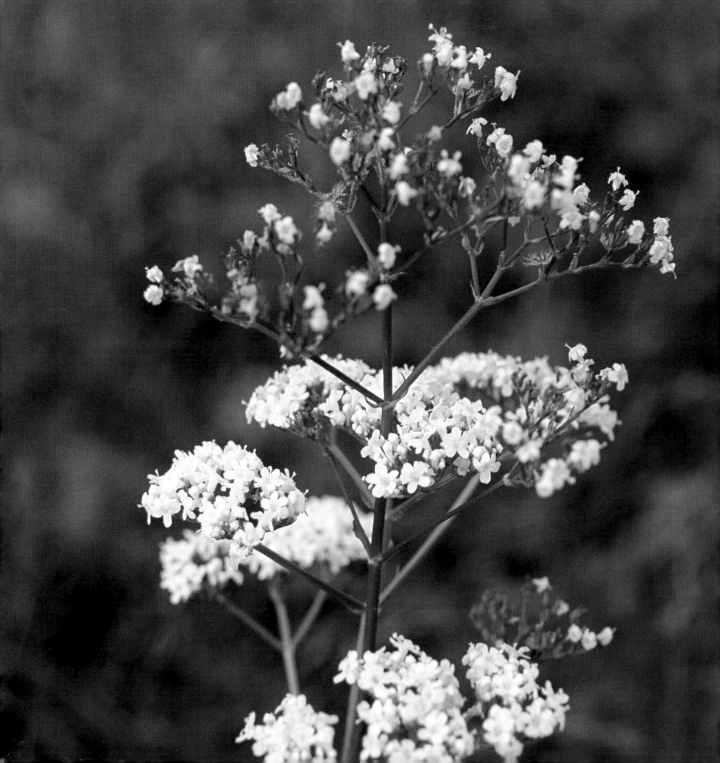

Chapter 3

Sleeping Well

Most of us are familiar with the sluggishness of our mental processes and the irritability that occurs after an extended period of wakefulness. Sleep restores normal levels of activity and balance in various aspects of the nervous system function. Sleep, or lack of sleep, has its direct effects on the central nervous system and not directly to muscles or organs; these are affected indirectly through the nervous system. Prolonged wakefulness is often associated with particular mental states such as anxiety and symptoms associated with imbalance of the nervous system.

During wakefulness, increased sympathetic activity occurs; during sleep, sympathetic activity decreases and parasympathetic activity increases. As a result of this nervous system shift during sleep, arterial blood pressure falls, pulse rate decreases, skin vessels dilate, activity of the gastrointestinal tract increases, muscles relax, and the overall rate of metabolism drops. If restful sleep does not occur, this shift does not occur and sympathetic activity remains high. Stimulating the sympathetic nervous system causes the release of epinephrine and norepinephrine (the hormones that are commonly thought of as adrenaline). These have a direct effect on muscle and liver cells, causing the release of stored energy and causing other increases in cellular activity. The shift toward sympathetic dominance at a time when sleep should occur generates energy and activity resulting in wakefulness. The food eaten during the day is not digested and absorbed properly; this means nutrition to every cell in the body decreases, impairing their optimal function. Skeletal muscles also do not relax, this inhibits the free flow of circulation in the body, again impairing cell function.

Other factors affecting sleep patterns are cortisol levels. Secretion of cortisol (a hormone secreted by the adrenal glands that releases energy) should be high in the morning and low in the evening. High levels promote wakefulness and give us energy; low levels support rest. High cortisol levels at night make it difficult to fall asleep, whereas low cortisol levels in the morning make it difficult to get up and cause a feeling of unrest. The adrenal response to prolonged stress is first to increase the output of cortisol, which leads to insomnia. Increased cortisol levels at night can alter rapid-eye movement (REM) and non-REM sleep cycles. Our understanding of the importance of REM sleep indicates that increased cortisol levels at night compromises the restorative and regenerative effects of a good night's sleep. Over an extended period, high cortisol levels diminish and, if unaddressed, eventually lead to adrenal exhaustion, resulting in chronic fatigue.

What Can You Do?

The ideal approach to sleeping well is not to rely on sleeping pills but to support restful sleep by balancing the nervous system and supporting the normal function of the adrenal glands, which produce cortisol and the neurotransmitters epinephrine and norepinephrine.

First, address the conditions in your life that cause stress to these systems and support your ability to respond to stress as discussed in Chapter 2. Then—and this is the most important change you can make to support the vibrant health of your nervous system and adrenal glands—completely stop or significantly decrease your consumption of caffeinated substances; these include coffee, black tea, chocolate, and cola. Green tea contains caffeine, but significantly less than black teas. Drinking green tea can be used as a transition when you stop drinking coffee or black tea. Herbal teas make excellent long-term substitutes for all these beverages. See Chapter 10 for the recipe for New Leaf Tea™, a supportive herbal tea to drink that will help you through the withdrawal phase as you eliminate caffeine.

Herbs can be used on an ongoing basis to support the adrenal glands and nervous system balance. Adaptogens and other adrenal modulators such as panax ginseng, Siberian ginseng, licorice root, oats,

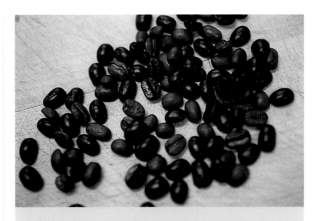

Caffeine is a drug that we can become dependent on. When we stop taking it, withdrawal symptoms such as severe headaches, irritability, restlessness, and fatigue can result.

and gotu kola help us adapt to or respond to stress. They are nourishing and balancing; they give us stamina and the ability to conserve energy. You will find these herbs used frequently throughout this book. Oats are featured in New Leaf Tea™ (Chapter 10) and Soothing Comfort Tea™ (Chapter 4), gotu kola is a primary ingredient in Simple Clarity™ herbal tea (Chapter 9), licorice root is featured in several teas including Immune Tonic Tea (Chapter 5), Liver Cleansing Tea (Chapter 7), and Lung Cleansing Tea (Chapter 8). Panax and Siberian ginseng are both very hard roots. If you use them to

Adaptogens include panax ginseng, Siberian ginseng, licorice root, oats, and gotu kola.

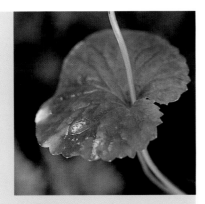

Gotu kola

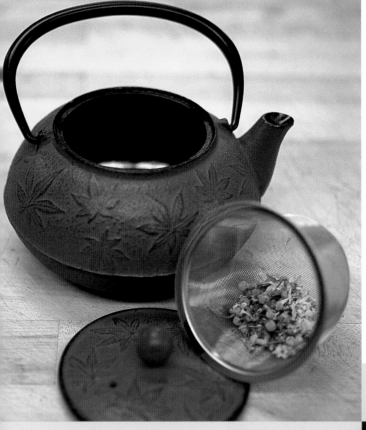

make a tea, they must be decocted (see the section on aqueous extractions in Chapter 13 for decocting instructions). They can also be quite stimulating and are therefore best taken in the morning and early afternoon; avoid taking the ginsengs after 2 PM.

Herbs such as those found in Sleep Well Tea restore nervous system balance, relax tight muscles, and act as a sedative.

Chamomile tea is probably the simplest and most easily accessible tea to make to facilitate a good night's sleep.

Valerian

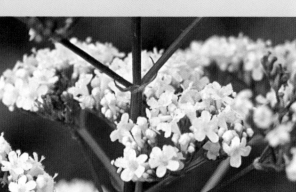

Sleep Well Tea

INGREDIENTS

> 1 teaspoon Valerian root
> 1 teaspoon Skullcap
> 1 teaspoon Passion flower
> 1-1/2 cups Almond milk
> Honey

INSTRUCTIONS

Place 1-1/2 cups pure cool water in a sauce pan. Add 1 heaping teaspoon of valerian root. Bring to a rolling boil and allow to simmer for 5 minutes. Add 1-1/2 cups almond milk and simmer another 5 minutes. Turn off the heat and add 1 heaping teaspoon skullcap herb and 1 heaping teaspoon passion flower. Let the mixture sit for another 5 minutes. Strain to remove the herbs, add honey to taste, and drink. Serves 2–3 people.

DOSE / TIMING / DURATION

Drink 1 cup half an hour before bed, sipping slowly.

BENEFITS

The sedative, relaxing to muscles and nerves, and antispasmodic qualities of these herbs make this a perfect after-dinner or before-bed beverage to calm digestive upset, ease you into sleep, and keep you soundly asleep all night long.

INDICATIONS

Insomnia, anxiety, nervous irritability, intestinal cramping, and muscle spasm.

CAUTIONS

- Valerian root and passion flower are known to increase the action of barbiturates.

- Passion flower should not be used during pregnancy because it contains uterine stimulants.

Herbal hydrotherapy is also a very effective tool for promoting sound sleep. See the Warming Sock Treatment and the Neutral Chamomile Bath presented here and the calming herbal baths in Chapter 11.

Warming Sock Treatment

The warming sock treatment is a simple, effective and time-honored tool that removes obstacles to healing and supports the body's ability to heal itself.

MATERIALS

1 pair of thick wool socks
1 pair of cotton socks
Lavender essential oil

INSTRUCTIONS

Immerse a pair of thin cotton socks in cold water. Sprinkle with a few drops of essential oil.

Soak your feet in a basin or tub of warm water for 5 to 10 minutes.

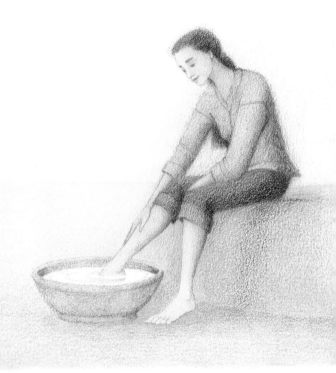

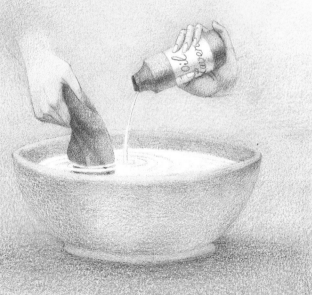

Wring the socks out thoroughly so they do not drip. Place the wet cotton socks on your feet. Then pull on the dry wool socks over them. Go directly to bed and keep yourself well covered.

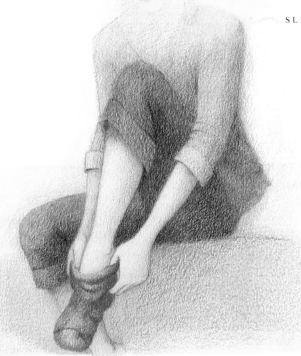

infections. The sock treatment also has a sedating action that facilitates a good night's sleep.

INDICATIONS

Sore throat, ear infections, headaches, nasal congestion, upper respiratory infections, coughs, bronchitis, colic, and insomnia.

CAUTIONS

This may not be appropriate for individuals with Raynaud's disease or other peripheral vascular diseases.

Your body will quickly generate heat to warm up your feet. If at any point during the treatment you find your feet getting chilled, give them a quick, brisk rub. Leave the socks on overnight. You will find that the cotton socks are dry in the morning.

DOSE / TIMING / DURATION

The warming sock treatment works best if it is repeated for three nights in a row. It is safe, and supportive, to use nightly.

BENEFITS

This soothing treatment gently stimulates the circulation and decreases congestion of the upper respiratory passages, head, and throat. It also relieves pain and stimulates the immune response, making it particularly useful during acute

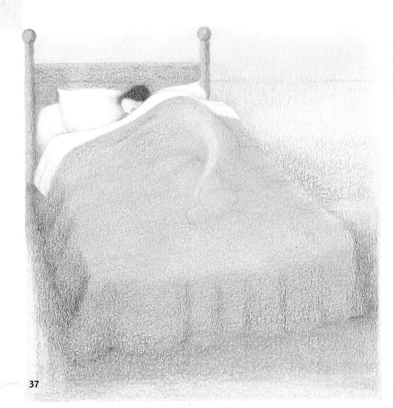

Neutral Chamomile Bath

MATERIALS

1/2 cup dried Chamomile flowers
Sock or gauze
Sheet or towels

INSTRUCTIONS

Place the chamomile flowers in a piece of gauze or in a sock and knot it at the end to make a little bag. Begin filling the bathtub with hot water, letting the water from the faucet fall onto your chamomile-filled bag. When the bath is approximately 1/4 full with the chamomile infusion, continue to fill the bathtub with cooler water. The goal is to finish with a bath that is body temperature, 94–97 degrees F. It is helpful to use a thermometer to achieve this temperature, but the most important guideline is how it feels to you. It should feel neither hot nor cold but, rather, neutral.

Immerse yourself in the neutral bath for at least 15 minutes and up to 1 hour. Cover any exposed body part (such as the knees) with a towel, or cover the entire bathtub with a sheet. At the end of the bath, cool the water slightly. Then get out of the tub, dry off quietly (excessive rubbing can disrupt the sedative effects), and go to bed.

DOSE / TIMING / DURATION

The neutral bath can be used nightly before bed, or when you wake in the middle of the night and have difficulty going back to sleep. It can also be used at other times of the day when calming and sedation is needed; in these cases, the bath should always be followed by at least 1/2 hour rest.

BENEFITS

Sedation, relief in congested areas due to equalization of circulation, tranquilization, and restoration of nervous balance.

INDICATIONS

Insomnia, nervous exhaustion, anxiety, and restlessness.

CAUTIONS

Long baths can be irritating to very dry or eczematous skin.

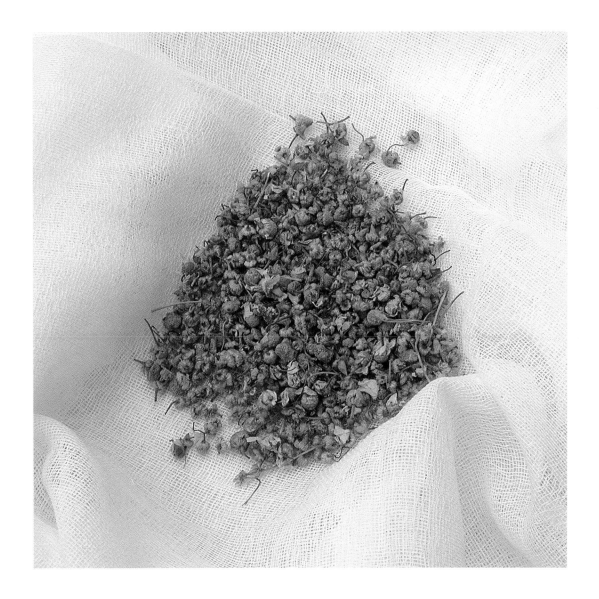

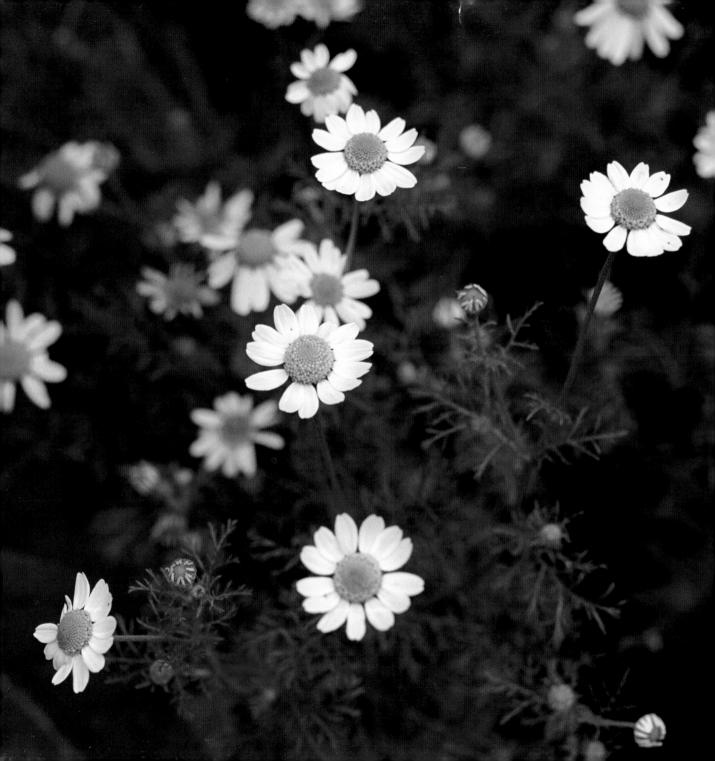

Chapter 4

The Key to Health: Efficient Digestion

Because the adverse health effects of poor nutrition, poor intake of nutrients, and poor absorption of nutrients are slow to be expressed as symptoms, we often do not associate our symptoms with digestion. Common symptoms such as fatigue, anxiety, depression, muscle cramps, poor memory, and difficulty concentrating can be caused by poor intake or assimilation of nutrients.

At the beginning of this book, I discuss health as a state of dynamic balance. We are in a constant interdependent exchange with our environment. In order to maintain homeostasis, the body is constantly taking in material from the environment, using what is nourishing, and eliminating material that is in excess or is harmful or toxic to the body. There are many organ systems through which the body interacts with its environment. Of these, I am tempted to say that the digestive tract is most important. But, of course, if the interaction between our environment and either the lungs or the kidneys were to decrease significantly life would end, so I cannot belittle their importance. Nevertheless, the digestive tract plays an extremely significant role that is often underestimated.

In order to function, every cell in our body requires specific nutrients. These nutrients are delivered to the cells via the blood, and they enter the bloodstream either as oxygen through the lungs or as food and fluids through the digestive tract. I think we minimize the importance of an optimally functioning digestive tract because its delivery process is a slow one. If we eat food that does not provide optimum nutrition, the resulting decreased function is not always apparent and is not immediately life threatening, unlike the functioning of the heart or brain. Yet the role of the digestive tract is at least as important; it is the way that cells acquire their life-sustaining nutrients—heart and brain cells included.

The Body's Largest Organ System

Our digestive tract is designed to achieve the slow absorption and assimilation of nutrients; it is the largest organ in the entire body. The small intestine alone is 20 feet in length and its surface area is magnified exponentially by the villi—the microscopic folds that make up the mucus lining of the digestive tract—and by the even more microscopic folds of each cell that lines the villi. The human body is an extremely efficient design, with multiple complex functions occurring in microscopic spaces, so for it to devote such a large area to digestion shows that the process must be important.

The digestive tract is a very long tube that starts with the mouth and ends at the anus. Along the way are a series of glands that secrete substances into the tube to facilitate various processes. These include the salivary glands, the liver and gallbladder, and the pancreas. The digestive tract also contains many types of immune-system cells that act as the body's defense against toxins entering through the digestive tract.

DIGESTION BEGINS IN THE MOUTH

You have been told about the importance of chewing your food, but it is something that is often overlooked in our fast-paced world. The act of chewing not only stimulates the flow of saliva, but it exposes the increasing surfaces of the food to the saliva. Covering the food with saliva lubricates the food so that it slips down the esophagus more readily and cools hot food to an appropriate temperature to reduce injury to the tender mucosal surface of the esophagus. Saliva production is regulated by the parasympathetic nervous system. This is stimulated by a sour taste, which is why foods such as vinegar or lemon are useful at the beginning of a meal. This aspect of the nervous system is inhibited by a stress response. When we eat while feeling afraid, nervous, or anxious, the body has more difficulty digesting the food.

THE STOMACH AND THE PARASYMPATHETIC NERVOUS SYSTEM

Food is mixed with gastric juices in the stomach, which mechanically breaks down the food. Gastric juice is made up of many substances including hydrochloric acid (HCl), which is crucial in the digestion of proteins; intrinsic factor needed for the absorption of Vitamin B-12 (a deficiency of which causes anemia); and enzymes that break down proteins, specifically those found in meats. The parasympathetic nervous system plays a role in relaxing the pyloric sphincter so that the food can leave the stomach and enter the duodenum.

Many people are deficient in HCl. One reason for this is that HCl secretion is stimulated by the parasympathetic nervous system, which decreases with the innervation of the sympathetic nervous system—the "fight or flight" response to stress. If we eat when we are stressed, the sympathetic nervous system is active, limiting the body's ability to secrete the needed HCl for healthy digestion. Proteins will be insufficiently broken down and will not move easily from the stomach into the duodenum.

REFLEXES OF DIGESTION

There is an intricate system of reflexes that coordinate movement of food through the digestive tract. The first reflex is called the duodenalcolic reflex. When the duodenum extends (that is when the stomach empties its contents into the duodenum), this causes a reflexive contraction in the colon—as if to signal, "There is more on its way, so we'd better make some room by emptying the colon." The second reflex is the gastroilial reflex. As the full stomach extends, the ileum (the final portion of the small intestine) contracts, moving its contents toward the colon. The third reflex is the enterogastric reflex. In this the distention of the small intestine sends an inhibitory signal to the stomach to slow down.

The amount of time that food stays in the stomach varies depending on the food. Fruits eaten alone move through the stomach in 20–30 minutes. Grains and vegetables take 1–2 hours, but a mixed meal, that is, one that contains foods from several different food groups, takes about 4 hours. Based on the reflex systems just described, we can see that it makes sense that we would have a bowel movement around the time that the stomach releases its contents into the duodenum, causing a reflexive contraction of the colon that results in elimination. We might deduce from this that in a healthy, optimally functioning digestive tract, we should have a bowel movement 2–4 hours after eating a meal. This means that three bowel movements daily could be considered normal function and that anything less would indicate a diminished function. In American culture,

I think, there is an idea that if you have a bowel movement once a day you are doing well—and compared to the many who have a bowel movement only every few days, this is true. However, one bowel movement a day may not indicate optimal health.

THE PANCREAS AND THE PARASYMPATHETIC NERVOUS SYSTEM

The pancreas secretes into the digestive tract substances that buffer the acid secretions of the stomach, multiple enzymes, and hormones such as insulin, somatostatin, and glucagon. Once again, the regulation occurs from the nervous system—parasympathetic stimulation increases the secretion of pancreatic enzymes, and sympathetic stimulation decreases pancreatic juices. One solution to direct digestive complaints, such as gas, bloating, and constipation, and indirect digestive complaints, such as fatigue, difficulty concentrating, and muscle spasms, is to take pancreatic enzymes. This will help, but it does not actually address the underlying cause of the problem—sympathetic dominance of the nervous system.

LIVER FUNCTIONS

The functions of the liver include the storage and filtration of the blood, overall metabolism, and formation of bile. Glucose, the sugar our cells need to function, is produced in the liver; energy is stored in the form of glycogen in the liver; and the synthesis of cholesterol (which is the backbone for all the steroidal hormones including estrogens, progesterone, and testosterone) occurs in the liver. The liver also converts carbohydrates and proteins to fat, forms the proteins that make up plasma, synthesizes amino acid, stores some vitamins including A, D, B-12, E, and K, stores iron in the form of ferritin, excretes drugs into bile for removal from the body, and alters or excretes hormones to maintain appropriate levels. The end products from metabolism in the liver are excreted via the bile to feces and via the serum, which is filtered in the kidneys and excreted in urine.

The liver therefore plays a crucial role in regulating the body's chemistry. The liver controls blood levels of cholesterol, fats, sugar, amino acids, and blood proteins. It is also the main organ of detoxification. Most foreign substances that enter the body via the mouth or the lungs, such as pollutants, prescription or recreational drugs, and food additives, are processed by the liver. Thus, in today's society where we are continually developing new chemicals and introducing them into our air, food, skin products, and so on, the liver is greatly overworked and often not functioning optimally.

Because the vitality of the liver impacts our health in so many ways, treatments for the liver are found throughout this book. For instance, hormonal imbalance may be a result of an accumulation of hormones in the blood due to a sluggish overburdened liver. Conditions of hormonal imbalance such as premenstrual syndrome (PMS) and peri-menopausal symptoms often respond, therefore, to herbs that support liver function; see Chapter 6 on hormonal balance for more details and specific therapies that support the liver's ability to balance hormones. Chapter 10 provides treatments that support breaking unhealthy addictions, in which, again, the liver can play an important role. At the end of this chapter, additional therapies are included that support the liver's role in creating vibrant skin and healthy joints and muscles.

SMALL INTESTINE

In the small intestine, the major absorption of carbohydrates, fats, and proteins occurs (the absorption of water occurs primarily in the large intestine). The stimulus for movement of food through the colon is the distention of the colon—this is why it is crucial to have fiber that creates bulk in the colon in the diet. Bulk equals distention, which stimulates movement.

Botanical medicines are generally liver friendly. In contrast to pharmaceutical drugs, which are a burden on the liver, most botanical medicines are easily metabolized and excreted by the liver. Alterative herbs are those that are balancing to gastrointestinal function. They enhance the absorption of nutrients, promote the elimination of wastes, and stimulate gastro-intestinal secretions, bile flow, and liver function. See the list of alterative herbs later in this chapter.

Tips to Optimize Digestion

- Eat or drink something tart or bitter before your meal to stimulate the flow of digestive juices. Apple cider vinegar or lemon can be used to make salad dressings—eat your salad before the rest of your meal. Bitter teas such as dandelion or skullcap make good before-meal drinks.

- Chew! Put your eating utensil down between bites and finish chewing the food completely before taking another bite.

- Don't drink with meals. Often liquids are used by people in lieu of proper chewing to wash food down. As a result, people miss not only the important mechanical breakdown of food but also the mixing of the food with saliva which, as already mentioned, begins the chemical breakdown of food and cools and lubricates the food so that it moves easily through the esophagus without damaging the delicate lining.

- Eat in a relaxed setting. Dim lights or candlelight help create a relaxing mood. Remember that digestion is powered by the parasympathetic nervous system, which is essentially inactivated when the sympathetic nervous system is triggered by stress. Having an argument while eating diminishes the body's ability to digest food and absorb nutrients from it. Our thoughts can also either support or diminish digestion. If we have a lot of negative feelings about the food we are about to eat, this will affect our ability to digest it. Eat with a feeling of joy and gratitude.

- Do not do other things while you eat. Turn off the TV and perhaps also the phone. Sit down when you eat. I have heard it said that it is better to eat a rock sitting down than the best food standing up. Today we should add "in the car or at your desk as you surf the Web."

Digestive Upsets

Because the body is in some phase of digestion most of the time, it is not only our mental and emotional state while we eat that impacts our digestion. Stress at any time will disrupt the digestive process. This can lead to chronic digestive problems such as constipation, which over time may lead to hemorrhoids, diverticular disease, or cancer of the colon. Poor digestion can lead to heartburn, gas, bloating, and cramping pain. The inhibition of the parasym-

pathetic nervous system means that there will be less digestive juices secreted throughout the digestive process, which means a diminished breakdown of foods, poor absorption of nutrients, and impaired elimination of metabolic wastes.

CARMINATIVE HERBS

Frequently experienced digestive complaints such as cramping pain, gas, and bloating can easily be addressed with herbs. Often these complaints are a result of overeating, eating too quickly, or eating when feeling stressed. In these circumstances, the symptoms can be relieved with herbs that are called carminatives. These include herbs such as chamomile, fennel, peppermint, oats, cinnamon, ginger, and lavender. These herbs can easily be infused, either individually or combined, to use as a tea. Tea is an ideal form for taking herbs that affect the digestive tract because it comes into direct contact with its mucosal lining. The Soothing Comfort Tea™ offered here works well for this purpose, as does New Leaf Tea™ offered in Chapter 10. You can also experiment on your own by trying any of the carminative herbs as a tea, individually or combined, when your intestines are cranky.

Soothing Comfort Tea™—A Digestive Tea

INGREDIENTS

1 part German Chamomile flowers
1 part Oats in milk
1 part Lavender buds
1 part Lemon balm leaf
1/8 part or to taste Stevia leaf

INSTRUCTIONS

Using your favorite tea-making tool (tea pot, French press, infusing basket, or tea ball), add a heaping teaspoon of herbs to each cup of just-boiled water. Cover and let sit for approximately 5 minutes. Pour the tea into a cup, straining out the herbs (or remove the infusing basket or tea ball), inhale the tea's aroma, and sip slowly.

DOSE / TIMING / DURATION

Drink up to 4 cups daily, as needed.

BENEFITS

These herbs act on the digestive tract and nervous system. They are anti-inflammatory, antispasmodic, pain relieving, and calming.

INDICATIONS

Digestive upset including cramping pain, bloating, flatulence, nervous exhaustion, stress, muscle tension, teething pain, headache, and insomnia.

CAUTIONS

- Chamomile may cause an allergic reaction in susceptible individuals, which may involve a skin rash, difficulty breathing, hives, or other hypersensitivity reactions. You should avoid chamomile if you know that you are allergic to plants in the Asteraceae/Compositae family. If you are unsure, introduce chamomile into your herbal repertoire carefully. If no adverse reaction occurs, you should feel free to use it freely.

- Lavender can bring on menses. Its extensive use should be avoided in the early stages of pregnancy.

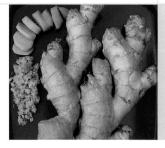

Carminative herbs include chamomile, fennel, peppermint, oats, cinnamon, ginger, and lavender.

Constitutional Hydrotherapy Self-Treatment

Also useful in the treatment of many digestive complaints is the constitutional hydrotherapy self-treatment. See Chapter 11 for administering hydrotherapy to others.

MATERIALS

2 wool blankets
1 sheet
1 towel
Shower or bath
Herbs for herbal infusion (See Table 2 on page 50)

INSTRUCTIONS

Prepare the bed first so that there is no delay between warming your body and being wrapped up. So begin by spreading the two wool blankets lengthwise on a bed; then cover the blankets with a sheet.

Soak a towel in a cold herbal infusion. If you do not have time to prepare an herbal infusion in advance, you can soak the towel in cold water to which you have added a few drops of essential oil.

Then take a nice hot shower or bath to warm up. Dry off. Wring the soaking towel out very well so that it does not drip, and then wrap it around your torso, covering the area from underneath your arms down to your pubic bone. Lay down on top of the sheet and blankets and wrap them around you. Now rest.

DOSE / TIMING / DURATION

Stay in the wrap for about 45 minutes or until the towel feels warmed. You can sleep, listen to quiet music, use visualization, or meditation. The treatment is best done daily. For chronic conditions, the treatment may be done daily for 3 weeks, followed by taking 1 week off, repeating the cycle again if necessary. For an acute condition such as a cold, it may be done daily for the duration of the condition. Often one hydrotherapy treatment at the first sign of an oncoming cold will ward off the cold completely.

BENEFITS

This is a deeply nourishing treatment that acts on a fundamental level to stimulate the body's self-healing mechanisms. It is a tonifying treatment; that is, it supports the most basic physiologic processes of digestion (assimilation of nutrients and detoxification of wastes), supports the immune system, relaxes muscles, and restores equilibrium to the nervous system. See Table 2 on next page.

INDICATIONS

This is a wonderful, simple home treatment for many acute and chronic health conditions, including digestive problems; respiratory conditions (but not acute asthma attacks), colds, and flu; PMS and menstrual pain; and muscle tension pain and soreness. See Table 2 on page 50.

CAUTIONS

- The treatment should not be used during an acute asthma attack, acute bladder infection, or rising fever.

- See Table 2 (page 50) for cautions for individual herbs.

Table 2

Herbs for Constitutional Hydrotherapy Treatment

HERBS	BENEFITS	INDICATIONS	CAUTIONS
Soothing Comfort Tea mixture:*Chamomile flowers, oatstraw, lavender buds, lemon balm leaf	Anti-inflammatory, antispasmodic, pain relieving, calming	Digestive upset including cramping pain, bloating, and flatulence; nervous exhaustion, stress, muscle tension, teething pain, headache, and insomnia	Chamomile may cause an allergic reaction in susceptible individuals.
Thyme	Expectorant, destroys bacteria	Congestion in the lungs accompanying a cold or flu	May cause irritation or allergic reaction in sensitive individuals.
Valerian root	Relieves muscle spasm, relaxing, sedating	Intestinal cramping, menstrual cramps, muscle pain and spasm, insomnia	Potentiates the action of barbiturates when taken internally.

* These herbs can also be used individually.

NOTES ON CONSTITUTIONAL HYDROTHERAPY SELF-TREATMENT

1. The point of the hot shower or bath is to warm the body before the application of cold. This can be accomplished in several other ways, including by exercising or spending 10 minutes in a sauna.

2. The application of the cold towel is therapeutic because it causes your body to generate warmth, increasing your circulation and metabolism. This is also when your body absorbs the water and herbs.

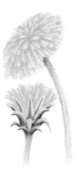

CONSTIPATION

Laxatives and Fiber

I have mentioned earlier that physiology indicates that we should have a bowel movement after each meal. In reality, people vary widely in the frequency of their bowel movements. Normal bowel habits can range from several per day to one every several days. To judge whether the bowels are constipated, we look to see whether there has been a decrease from a person's normal frequency and if there is difficulty passing the stools. Straining, pain, and size of the stool (such as small hard balls instead of a large well-formed mass) are probably the best indicators of a problem.

There are several approaches to the treatment of constipation. One of the most common is the use of bulk laxatives, usually Metamucil or "fiber" capsules. Instead of this, it is better to get this fiber directly by eating whole grains, such as brown or red rice and oatmeal. Equally important is regular intake of water-soluble fibers such as those found in juicy fruits and vegetables. It is commonly recommended that people eat 5–6 servings of fruits and vegetables per day. Another approach offered is 80% of our food intake should be fruits and vegetables; the other 20% should be concentrated foods such as proteins, starches, and fats.

The other kind of laxative is an irritant laxative, commonly available in the supermarket. These soften and expel the stool quickly. The most commonly used herbal irritant laxative is senna. The use of senna or other irritant laxatives on occasion is all right, but regular use of them instead of the fibers just discussed can cause problems. Habitual use of laxatives will sidestep the body's natural processes for producing a bowel movement, leading to a dependence on the laxative. If constipation is chronic and does not respond to dietary changes such as increasing dietary fiber and water intake, an investigation with a healthcare practitioner is indicated to rule out a potentially life-threatening cause.

Alterative Herbs

Alteratives are wonderful herbs that support digestion in many ways and that also have a mild laxative effect. Some are bitter herbs that promote the flow of digestive juices, gently improving natural physiological functioning and supporting digestion, the absorption of nutrients, and the elimination of wastes. Unlike irritant laxatives, the alteratives can be used over an extended period of time—in fact, they are best used over an extended period of time. They generally will not have an immediate effect on elimination (although they do for some individuals), but the quality and frequency of bowel movements will generally respond to alteratives after several weeks. Some alteratives useful for constipation are dandelion, Oregon grape, and yellow dock. See Liver Cleansing Tea in Chapter 7 for a good alterative tea that will help relieve constipation.

HEARTBURN

Heartburn is a burning pain underneath the sternum, or breastbone, that rises in the chest and may radiate or spread out to the neck, throat, or face. Two major causes of heartburn are gastroesophageal reflux disease (GERD) and hypochlorhydria. Heartburn usually occurs after meals, especially when a person is lying down. It may be accompanied by a regurgitation of stomach contents into the esophagus.

Gastroesophageal Reflux Disease

Heartburn may be accompanied by GERD (reflux of the stomach contents into the esophagus). The esophagus is normally protected by the lower

Alterative herbs for constipation include dandelion, Oregon grape, and yellow dock.

esophageal sphincter, and the downward motion of peristalsis. Disruption of either of these leads to reflux. The esophageal sphincter is weakened by coffee and caffeine, smoking, alcohol, fats, chocolate, mint, and pregnancy. Right after eating, lying down can interrupt the downward motion of peristalsis and deep forward-bending movements can force the stomach contents back upward.

Natural protection against heartburn is also provided by the alkalinizing effect of swallowing saliva. This underlines, again, the importance of chewing. If we do not chew, we do not secrete as much saliva and do not mix it with our food as it travels downward, and we lose its alkalinizing effects. The simplest remedy is, of course, to remove the aggravating factors such as frequent coffee consumption and use of breath mints and to not eat for 2–3 hours before lying down.

An additional, and these days most common, cause of heartburn is the use of Tums or other over-the-counter antacid. Although over-the-counter antacids may temporarily reduce the sensation of burning, over time they exacerbate the condition. Tums is calcium carbonate. In order to absorb calcium carbonate, the body must produce acid, so taking in calcium carbonate actually leads to an increase in stomach acid rather than a decrease.

Do you have heartburn? Avoid peppermint tea and breath mints. Peppermint tea is almost a cure-all because of its many beneficial uses, many of which are digestive. Heartburn, however, is *not* one of them. All types of mint have the potential of relaxing the lower esophageal sphincter and causing a reflux of gastric contents.

Hypochlorhydria

The sensation of heartburn is not always the result of too much stomach acid; in fact, in most cases it is the opposite—a symptom of decreased stomach acid, or hypochlorhydria. The pain can actually be an alkaline burn from the duodenum or stomach, and taking antacid medications will only exacerbate this problem.

The causes of hypochlorhydria include autoimmune disease, *Helicobactor pylori* infection, regular consumption of processed foods, excess fat and sugar intake, chronic overeating, hypothyroidism,

DIGESTIVE TONIC

Make a vinegar of dandelion leaf, gentian, and skullcap (see Chapter 13 on making your own medicines). You may choose to use all three of these herbs to make your digestive tonic, a combination of two of them, or simply one of them. Use the Herb Index to help make the most appropriate choices for you.

Ways to take the digestive tonic:

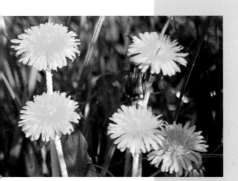

- Place 1 tablespoon in room-temperature water in the morning upon rising. Sip slowly. This will quench your early morning thirst, stimulate digestion so that your body is really ready for breakfast, and be invigorating—you may find that it easily replaces your early morning dose of caffeine in the form of coffee, tea, or cola.

- Take 1 tablespoon in water 15–20 minutes before every meal.

- Add 1 tablespoon to a cup of warm or hot water with 1 tablespoon of organic honey to make a delicious warm beverage.

- If you carry a water bottle with you in your car or on a hike, add 1 tablespoon to this water and sip it throughout the day. You will find it to be thirst quenching and revitalizing. *Beware:* The acidity of vinegar can leach toxins from light plastic containers into your water. A glass container is preferable, but, if you must use plastic, heavy plastic is better than the lightweight clear plastic of most water bottles.

hypoadrenalism, chronic stress, and salt-restricted diets. Disease states that have been associated with hypochlorhydria include childhood asthma, hypothyroidism, hyperthyroidism, eczema, gall bladder inflammation or stones, rheumatoid arthritis, urticaria, lupus erythematosis, adrenal exhaustion, chronic hepatitis, chronic gastritis, vitiligo, and rosacea. If you know that you have one of these conditions and you have heartburn or other digestive problems, hypochlorhydria may be a contributing factor. Hypochlorhydria can cause a malabsorption of nutrients that can manifest in almost any system, causing anemia, depression, fatigue, muscle spasm, hormonal imbalances, and so on.

To treat this condition:

- Take apple cider vinegar (1 tablespoon in warm water) before each meal or consider a trial of herbally infused apple cider vinegar to see if it makes a difference (see the Digestive Tonic recipe). (Note: Hydrochloric acid supplementation is often recommended, but I suggest taking apple cider vinegar before meals instead. Fresh-squeezed lemon juice in water also serves this purpose for many people.)

- Develop tools for dealing with stress. As you do so, you will be less likely to overeat and you will begin to eat only when you are actually hungry.

- Take short, strolling (not vigorous) walks after eating. The muscle activity produces acids that decrease the need for the cells of the stomach to conserve acid.

- Avoid excessive intake of dietary sugars and fats.

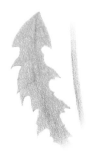

IRRITABLE BOWEL SYNDROME

Irritable bowl syndrome (IBS), also called spastic colon, may manifest as abdominal pain, constipation or diarrhea or both, mucus in stools, gas, nausea, anxiety, or depression. It is aggravated by stress and a low-fiber diet. Treatment includes stress reduction, elimination of food allergies, and a high-fiber diet. Herbal treatments can include licorice, fennel, chamomile or peppermint, as tea either individually or by mixing two or more together. Also, slippery elm as a gruel or tea will soothe an irritated digestive tract.

Slippery Elm Gruel

INGREDIENTS

1-1/2 teaspoon powdered Slippery elm bark
1/4 cup cold Water or juice
1-1/2 cups boiling Water or juice (apple or grape tastes great)
Honey or maple syrup, raisins, lemon rind, cinnamon, cloves, nutmeg or other spices

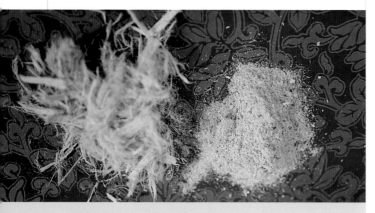

SLIPPERY ELM TEA

Bring water to a rolling boil, add 1 teaspoonful of finely cut slippery elm bark for every cup of water. Let simmer for 5 minutes. Strain out the herb. Drink 3–4 cups of tea per day.

INSTRUCTIONS

Mix powdered slippery elm bark with 1/4 cup of cold water or juice to make a paste. Stirring steadily, pour 1-1/2 cups of boiling water or juice into the paste and continue stirring for 2 minutes with a spoon. To this basic gruel, you can add honey or maple syrup, raisins, lemon rind, or spices.

DOSE / TIMING / DURATION

Take 1–2 cups one to three times per day.

BENEFITS

This contains considerable mucilage, starch, sugars, tannins, and trace minerals. It is used as a demulcent (soothes inflamed or damaged tissue) and nutritive tonic.

INDICATIONS

Internally, it is primarily used to soothe irritated or inflamed mucous membranes of the respiratory and gastrointestinal tract. This includes sore throats, coughs, bronchitis, pneumonia, gastritis, ulcers, colitis, and diarrhea. It can be used as a food source and nutritive tonic during acute and recovery stages of healing.

CAUTIONS

Dried slippery elm bark should always be taken with water.

Digestion and Clear Vibrant Skin

The liver is the body's primary organ of detoxification. When the liver becomes overburdened, the other organs of detoxification—the lungs, kidneys, bowels, and skin—have to work harder to keep up with the cleansing needs of the body.

Toxins are eliminated from the body through the skin, primarily by sweating and by the regular sloughing off of skin cells. When other organs of elimination are not functioning optimally, we see skin conditions—acne, eczema, and other rashes—arise as the skin tries to compensate. If we suppress these skin eruptions, we are further hindering the body's effort to rid itself of toxins. We have not addressed the problem and are likely to experience more symptoms down the road—perhaps more skin problems, or perhaps more serious conditions.

Thus, when we see acne, eczema, and other skin eruptions we should think about cleansing the liver to support adequate elimination through the digestive tract. By cleansing the liver we are taking the excess burden off the skin, and the eruptions generally resolve. So our first herbs in treating skin conditions are liver- and bowel-cleansing herbs.

Digestion and Healthy Joints and Muscles

Many things influence joint health: posture, body weight, types of activities, bone density, heredity, diet, the amount of fluids taken in, the health of the digestive system, the degree of the body's toxic burden, and the balance of body chemistry. All these factors must be considered and possibly addressed to relieve joint pain. The mechanical issues listed are not within the scope of this book, but they are crucial elements. They can be addressed beautifully with yoga and perhaps some kind of body work. We focus here on the issues of digestive health, minimizing the toxic burden on the body, and balancing body chemistry. The liver plays a role here, too.

Osteo-arthritis is known to be caused by wear and tear on the joints. It is characterized by a degeneration of the cartilage where the ends of two bones meet. The liver produces substances that stimulate the production of cartilage cells. If the liver is congested, it has a difficult time accomplishing this, as well as its many other functions.

Bowel health and joint inflammation are also related. In Ayurvedic medicine, a 5,000-year-old system from India, arthritis is considered to be caused

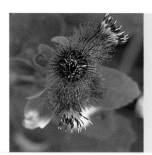

Burdock

Clear Skin Tea

INGREDIENTS

1 part Burdock root
1 part Yellow dock root
1 part Oregon grape root
1/2 part Ginger root, cinnamon bark, or
    orange peel (optional for flavor)

INSTRUCTIONS

Place pure cool water in a sauce pan and add 1 tablespoon of the herb mixture for every cup of water. Bring to a rolling boil. Allow the herbs to simmer for 10 minutes. Turn off the heat and let sit for another 5 minutes. Strain out the herbs and drink the remaining liquid.

DOSE / TIMING / DURATION

Drink 3–4 cups per day. These herbs are tonics for the body and can be used safely on an ongoing basis.

BENEFITS

Supports the elimination of metabolic wastes through the liver and supports the digestive and lymphatic systems, so the skin does not have to do all the work. These are multifunction herbs that are liver cleansing and have a specific affinity for the skin.

INDICATIONS

Acne, eczema, psoriasis, boils, carbuncles, and sties.

CAUTIONS

- Oregon grape root and burdock should not be used during pregnancy because they contain several compounds that stimulate the uterus.

- Yellow dock should be used cautiously by individuals with a history of oxalate kidney stones.

- Remember that it is a good idea to take "vacations" from any herb that you use regularly. Consider taking a 2-week break every 3–4 months.

by toxic colon. Cleansing herbs and diet can be used to restore healthy function of the digestive tract and liver, which in turn affects the joints, increasing mobility and decreasing pain. In my Naturopathic practice, I frequently see joint pains go away following dietary changes that reduce inflammation and support the liver. See the Liver Cleansing Tea in Chapter 7.

You can decrease inflammation by ingesting essential fatty acids (EFAs) such as flax, borage oil and evening primrose oil. The essential fatty acids in these herbs inhibit the production of inflammatory prostaglandins in the body. These oils are readily available in health food stores. Make sure they are unrefined and packaged in dark bottles. These oils are very fragile and are destroyed easily by heat. They must be stored in the refrigerator and should never

SUPER SALAD DRESSING

Ingredients:
- 1 teaspoon Dijon mustard
- 2 tablespoons Apple cider vinegar
- 1/2 cup extra virgin Olive oil
- 1 tablespoon Flax oil
- 1 teaspoon fresh herbs or 1 clove crushed garlic (optional)

Dip a fork into the jar of mustard and transfer about 1 teaspoon to a small bowl. Add vinegar and mix. Add olive oil in a thin stream while stirring with the fork until the oil is well emulsified. Add flax oil and herbs. Use immediately.

(This recipe is based on recipes in Sally Fallon's book *Nourishing Traditions,* an excellent resource for truly healthy home cooking.)

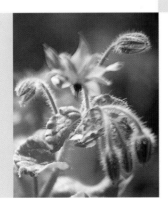

Borage flowers, including the seeds, which contain the valuable fatty acids, can be eaten whole. Add borage flowers to spring and summer salads.

be cooked. Add these oils to your foods after they have been cooked or use them along with olive oil to make your own salad dressing.

Topical remedies for joint pain, stiff or sore muscles, and inflammation are included in Chapter 12.

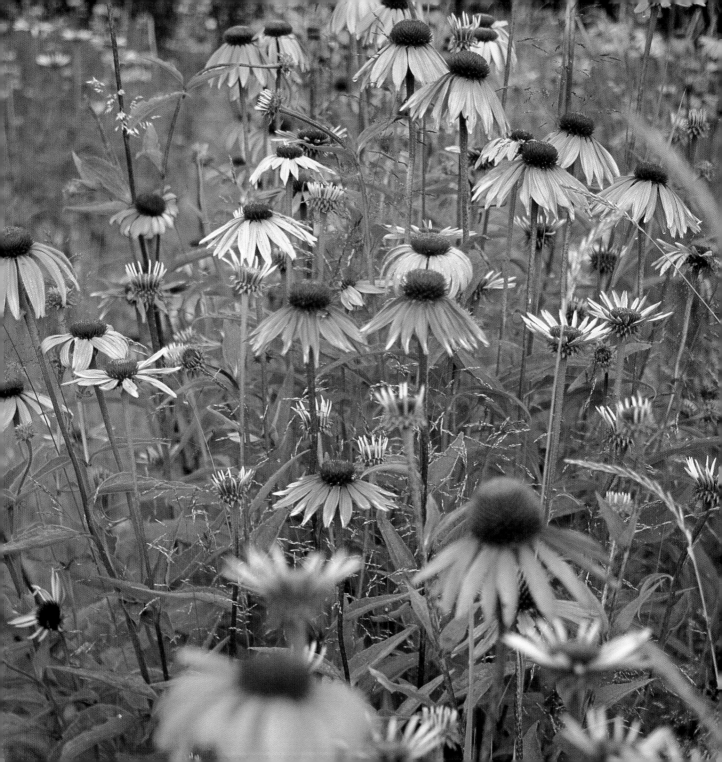

Chapter 5

Strong Immunity

As we find ourselves facing ever more virulent viruses and bacteria (including those that have become resistant to antibiotics) and a steadily increasing rise in the incidence of all types of cancers, the need for a strong immune system is at last becoming apparent. In the twentieth century, we bought into the idea that microbes are the cause of disease and poured our resources into the development of drugs to kill these microbes. In doing this, we took our attention away from our personal responsibility for creating our state of wellness. We ignored the hospitable environment in our body that allows these invading pathogens or (in the case of cancer) abnormal cells to survive and even thrive. To live a life not plagued by one cold after another or to not be the one of every three people diagnosed with cancer, we must take steps to optimize the function of the immune system.

The immune system is a little hard to describe anatomically because it is not a series of structures like the digestive tract and the cardiovascular system. With a few exceptions, the immune system is microscopic. There are cells all over the body with immune functions. There are many different kinds of cells, each with a specific role in defending the body from foreign invaders. There are cells that attach themselves to invading pathogens such as viruses and essentially call out to the immune cells that devour the intruder to come and get it. A foreign invader can be much more than just viruses and bacteria. Our bodies come into contact with all sorts of substances that are unfamiliar to it and that the immune system then needs to take care of. We are constantly creating more and more new substances, from hybridized foods to chemicals, food dyes, preservatives, pharmaceutical drugs, and plastics that we cook in and eat from—all of which we take in to our bodies. Because these substances are so numerous, the immune system can become overly taxed and overwhelmed, and we begin to feel ill. It is then that abnormal function can take advantage of the immune system's being busy and take over. Cancer is

a good example of this. It is most likely that abnormal cell growth occurs in humans on a regular basis. The immune system spots these abnormal growths and stops them before they get out of control. But if foreign substances overwhelm the immune system, abnormal cell growth could go unchecked. This speaks to doing everything we can to decrease the burden on the immune system and, of course, do whatever we can to support healthy function of these cells every day, not just after we become ill.

Immune Depressors

As I mentioned earlier, stress plays a large role in depressing immune function. Managing stress and other lifestyle factors such as getting adequate rest and ensuring the adequate intake and absorption of certain vitamins and minerals are known to support healthy immune function. The following are known to depress the immune system.

- Stress
- Inadequate sleep
- Sugar intake
- Exposure to allergens (food and environmental)

- Toxic buildup (not enough cleansing through bowels, lungs, and kidneys)

- Trans fats intake

- Coffee intake

- Tobacco smoking

When intake or exposure to these stressors is extreme or frequent, the immune system becomes overwhelmed and the simple steps needed to maintain a healthy immune system may no longer be enough to restore balance. Immune supportive herbs taken as teas, as tinctures, or in capsules play an important role at this stage.

Immune Supportive Diet

Dietary habits are absolutely critical to maintaining strong immunity. The ingestion of certain foods such as sugar is known to depress immune function, while foods such as fruits, vegetables, legumes and whole grains are filled with nutrients that make it strong. As a general rule, eat more fruits and vegetables—as much as you can. Don't stress about it because stress will inhibit your ability to digest the food and absorb the nutrients.

Just choose colorful produce to eat whenever you can.

As I mention in Chapter 4, some dietary programs suggest that 80% of all the food you eat should be vegetables and fruit, with the other 20% being concentrated foods such as proteins and starches. Dark green foods contain chlorophyll, which is anti-carcinogenic, so eat dark greens such as kale, collards, bok choy, dandelion, mustard greens, beet greens, and fresh nettles from your garden at least once a day.

Yellow, orange, and red foods are high in carotenoids and anti-oxidants. They enhance white blood cell activity and promote the function of many immune system cells. Foods in the crucifer family are probably the best-known anti-cancer foods. These include broccoli, cabbage, cauliflower, mustard greens, Brussels sprouts, radishes, and turnips. Herbs that strengthen the immune system by providing chlorophyll and other essential nutrients should be included in your diet; some of these deeply nourishing green plants are:

- Nettles—can be steamed or used in any cooked dish in which you would use spinach

- Chickweed—delicious added to salads

- Alfalfa—as sprouts, a live, cleansing, and nourishing

Oregon grape is an effective and ecologically and economical substitute for the popular herb goldenseal. Until recently, goldenseal was not cultivated; it was harvested from the wild as a cold and flu remedy. Because of its growing popularity, this led to its overharvesting and to its near-extinction, raising the price of goldenseal considerably. Organic farmers have begun to cultivate goldenseal recently; however, it takes several years to develop a crop with mature roots ready for harvesting. Oregon grape contains many of the same alkaloids as goldenseal including berberine (the old name for Oregon grape or mahonia was berberis) and is much more readily available. Oregon grape grows quite prolifically in many different environments.

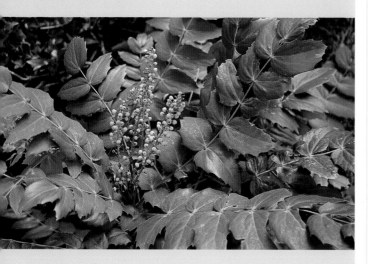

Mahonia nervosa, a low-growing shade-loving variety of Oregon grape.

food that can be added to your salads or used in sandwiches in place of lettuce

- Dandelion leaf—as fresh spring greens, add to your salads

The word tonic in the Immune Tonic Tea recipe on the next page indicates that the herbs in it are supportive of the body's basic physiological process; they strengthen the body's self-healing mechanism. These herbs are ones that you might drink regularly throughout the cold and flu season to keep yourself healthy.

Fighting Colds and Flu

Frequent colds and flu indicate that the immune system is weak. This chapter includes a number of things you can do to strengthen your immunity before you become susceptible to more serious or chronic immunosuppressive conditions.

The time to take action is when you first have an inkling that you might be getting sick. At this point, you can actually keep the cold or flu from coming on by taking immediate action. The early warning signs may be a scratchy throat, an achy tired feeling, or that feeling of just not quite being up to par. This is the point when the metaphoric glass of water is

Immune Tonic Tea

INGREDIENTS

1 part Astragalus root
1 part Burdock root
1 part Oregon grape root
1 part Dandelion root
1/2 part Licorice root
1/2 part Orange peel

INSTRUCTIONS

Place pure cool water in a sauce pan and add 1 tablespoon of the herb mixture for every cup of water. Bring to a rolling boil. Allow the herbs to simmer for 10 minutes. Turn off the heat and let sit for another 5 minutes. Strain out the herbs and drink the remaining liquid.

DOSE / TIMING / DURATION

Drink 1–4 cups daily. This can be taken on a regular basis to support immunity or during times of increased stress on the immune system, such as loss of sleep or pushing to meet deadlines.

BENEFITS

This immune tonic tea consists of herbs that are both cleansing (decreasing the body's burden) and immune system supportive (nourishing and strengthening the self-healing mechanism). The herbs also have anti-viral, anti-bacterial, and anti-inflammatory properties.

INDICATIONS

Chronically depressed immunity, weakness, fatigue, and busy stressful times when a little extra support is needed to fend off illness.

CAUTIONS

Oregon grape root should not be used during pregnancy because it contains several compounds that stimulate the uterus. If you are pregnant, make this tea without the Oregon grape root.

IMMUNE SUPPORTIVE TEA

To supplement the benefits of the green plants in your diet I highly recommend using deep nourishing greens as teas. These are some of the most nourishing plants on the planet and are not found in the everyday American diet. Teas are a great way to include herbs such as nettles, red raspberry leaf, chickweed, cleavers, and dandelion in your diet.

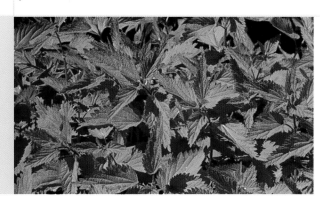

brimming but has not yet begun to overflow. At this point, if you carefully remove some of the water from the glass, it will not overflow at all—that is, you can keep the cold symptoms from ever manifesting. Sometimes all that is needed to keep the glass from

overflowing is to change one of the contributors to the weakened immune system. But the glass is still quite full, so the next stress to come along will tend to bring it back up to the top and perhaps overflow it into symptoms. What is generally required at this point, when your body is on the brink of illness, is to empty the glass of water—that is, to decrease the burden on your body in as many ways as you can to cleanse the body of its toxic load.

The way to decrease the burden on the body from a dietary standpoint is to eat lightly and to focus on foods that are cleansing and that the body can digest easily, such as rice, steamed vegetables, soups, and salads. Very often when we are under a lot of stress, the first thing to go out the window is a healthy diet. We start to eat convenient fast food or comfort foods, all of which add to the body's burden, taking the body out of balance. Herbs that support the immune system, such as onions, garlic, Shitake mushrooms, and burdock root, can be added to soup to enhance its immune system supportive properties. Eating soup, then, serves two purposes: to decrease the burden on the body (lowering the level of water in the glass) and to strengthen the immune system to allow the body to heal itself. See recipe on page 69 for Immune Supportive Soup.

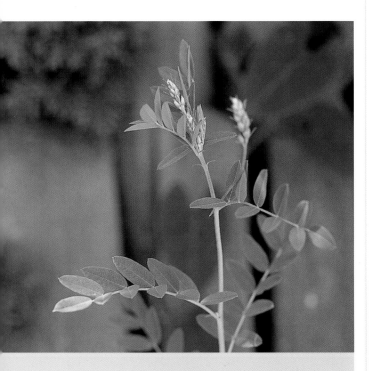

Astragalus

Shitake mushrooms are effective immune potentiators.

The next thing to do is get rest as soon as possible. Many people ignore the early warning signs of illness and keep working until they drop. You will take longer to heal if you allow the illness to get a foothold. If you feel a sore throat, headache, or congestion coming on, take it easy. If possible, take a day off from work. This may prevent you from having to take three days off later on.

Also, drink plenty of fluids. This standard advice is good advice. You can clear toxins from your system with large amounts of filtered water and herb teas. Contrary to common thought, juices are not the ideal fluids for immune system support. Juice has a lot of sugar, which depresses immunity. Eating whole fruit is better than drinking juice because it still has the fiber intact, which means the sugar moves into the bloodstream more slowly and because you consume a more moderate amount of sugar in a piece of fruit than in a cup of juice (which contains the sugar from many pieces of fruit). Orange juice, in particular, increases mucus production in many individuals—mucus provides a hospitable environment for microbes to live and multiply. If you are going to drink juices as part of your fluid intake during a cold, it is best to dilute the juices by half—50% water, 50% juice. A fabulous alternative to orange juice is freshly squeezed carrot and beet juices, perhaps with a little fresh apple or ginger.

Garlic and onions stimulate the white blood cells and are anti-bacterial, anti-viral, and anti-fungal.

Kelp is a sea vegetable that is very rich in iodine, which stimulates the thyroid and metabolism in general. Many kinds of kelp have been seen to inhibit cancer growth in laboratory studies, and may stimulate T-cell production. Seaweeds are generally very salty in taste and can be used as a salt replacement.

Teas are very useful in fighting colds. Just the warmth of the tea helps open up congested passageways and soothe your system. The Immune Tonic Tea given on page 65 is perfect for fighting colds. Another excellent immune system supportive tea is Echinacea Lemon Ginger Tea™ on page 70. This contains the very popular immune stimulant echinacea. Ginger is a warming herb that potentiates the action of echinacea.

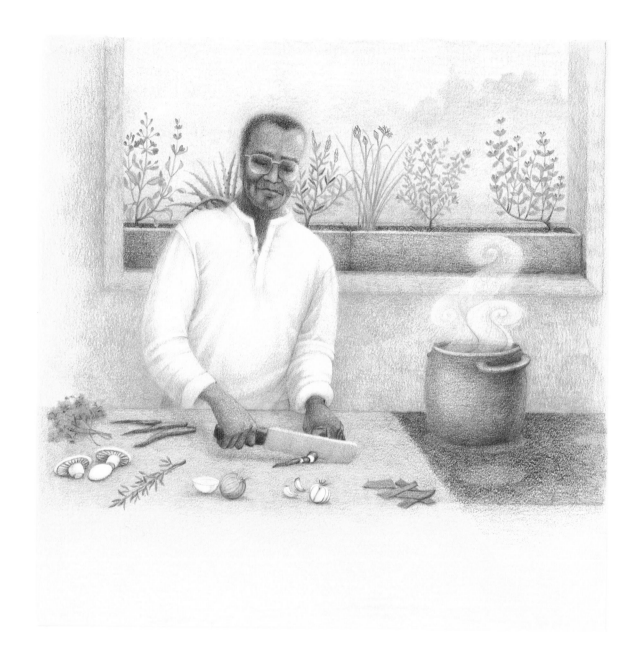

Immune Supportive Soup

INGREDIENTS

Olive oil
10 cups Water
1 large Onion
3–5 large Garlic cloves
1 cup Celery
1 cup Shitake mushroom
1 teaspoon Black pepper
2 Potatoes
1/2 teaspoon Cayenne pepper
1 inch Ginger root
1/2 cup your choice of fresh herbs, such as
    fresh parsley, rosemary, thyme, oregano,
    and fennel
3 Astragalus sticks (if finely cut astragalus is
    used, wrap it in cheese cloth, tie it closed
    with a string, and add to the soup)
4 large Carrots
2 large Burdock root
1/2 cup dried Kelp

INSTRUCTIONS

Sauté the onion and garlic in a little olive oil. Add 10 cups pure water and bring to a boil. Add vegetables and simmer covered for 1 hour. Add the herbs for the last 10 minutes. Strain out the astragalus root and serve.

DOSE / TIMING / DURATION

You can use this immune soup as your primary food source when your appetite is suppressed during an acute cold or flu, eating a bowl three or four times a day until your appetite returns, signaling that the body can easily process heavier foods. The soup can also be consumed any time you wish to give your immune system a little support.

BENEFITS

This soup provides nutrients to the body in a form that it can easily digest and absorb. The energy of the body is not diverted away from its job of protecting the body from invading pathogens to process foods that require a lot of energy to digest. The ingredients stimulate white blood cell activity as well as destroying or suppressing the growth of bacteria, viruses, and fungi.

INDICATIONS

At first sign of a cold or flu, any time you are feeling run down, overworked, or depleted, or as a regular part of your diet to maintain a strong defense system. Try having this soup for breakfast instead of eggs and toast or cereal. It can easily be made, stored in the refrigerator, and then eaten over several days. Or make a large batch and freeze it in individual-size serving containers that can easily be thawed and reheated as desired.

CAUTIONS

There are no general cautions or contra-indications to consuming this soup. A food such as this is the safest way to use herbs. If you take pharmaceutical medications such as blood thinners, it is possible that your need for the medication will diminish with regular consumption of herbs such as garlic. In this case, regular monitoring by your healthcare practitioner is indicated.

Echinacea Lemon Ginger Tea™— An Immune Support Tea

INGREDIENTS

1 part *Echinacea purpurea* whole plant
1/2 part *Echinacea angustifolia* root
1 part Ginger root
3/4 part Orange peel
3/4 part Lemon grass
1/4 part Lemon peel
1/8 part Stevia leaf

INSTRUCTIONS

Using your favorite tea-making tool (tea pot, French press, infusing basket, or tea ball), add a heaping teaspoon of the herb mixture to each cup of just boiled water. Cover and let sit for approximately 5 minutes. Pour the tea into a cup, straining out the herbs (or remove the infusing basket or tea ball), inhale the tea's aroma, and sip slowly.

DOSE / TIMING / DURATION

Begin drinking this tea at first sign of a cold and continue to drink 4–8 cups per day for up to 1 week or until symptoms subside. If symptoms worsen, do not respond to home therapies, are accompanied by a high fever, or continue for more than 3 weeks, it is important to consult with a healthcare provider. For sore throats, gargle with the echinacea tea before swallowing.

BENEFITS

The immune-system-supporting, anti-viral, and anti-bacterial properties of echinacea are well known. Ginger is the perfect synergist for echinacea because its warming properties potentiate the action of the echinacea. Ginger also promotes sweating and expectoration (both avenues of elimination)—perfect for the treatment of colds and flu. This is a pleasant-tasting tea, making it easy to drink it frequently throughout an acute illness.

INDICATIONS

This tea is different than the Immune Tonic Tea. Echinacea is most effective when used at first sign of an illness, not as a long-term preventative. Prepare this tea when you first begin to notice signs of illness. Taken at that time it will either prevent the cold from taking hold or it will shorten the length of the illness or decrease its severity. This tea is specifically indicated when there is lymphatic congestion and swollen glands.

CAUTIONS

There is no known toxicity associated with either short- or long-term use of echinacea. There is some belief that it loses its effectiveness with long-term use, but this is not proven clearly to be the case. Individuals with auto-immune diseases or AIDS should consult a healthcare practitioner familiar with the use of herbs before including echinacea as a regular part of their health maintenance program.

GARGLING WITH HERBS

For sore throats, gargling with an herbal extract is highly effective because of the direct contact of the herbs with the affected surfaces. You can simply gargle with an echinecea tea or tincture before swallowing it. Propolis also makes a very effective sore throat gargle. To use a propolis extract purchased from a natural foods store, place 30 drops of propolis in a small amount of water, gargle, and swallow.

PROPOLIS EXTRACT

Propolis extract can easily be made by placing an alcohol and water mixture (65–95% alcohol) over propolis acquired from a local beekeeper (see Chapter 13 for information on making tinctures and other extracts). The propolis will dissolve leaving a thick extract.

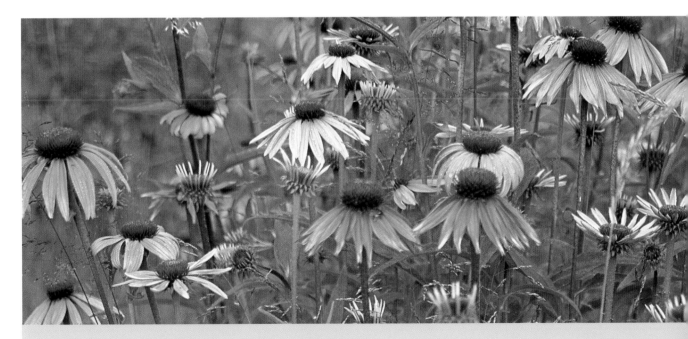

Echinacea

DETOXIFICATION

Another crucial element in decreasing the body's burden is to promote detoxification in as many ways as possible, for example, by sweating from exercise, a sauna, or the Bath and Sweat described in Chapter 8. Deep breathing supports the elimination of toxins through the lungs. Deep breathing can be stimulated by exercise or, if you are unable to exercise, you can simply sit up in bed and lengthen the exhalation repeatedly until your breathing expands. Try taking a deep breath in through your nose and exhaling through your mouth with a loud whisper of the syllable "ha" until all the breath has been exhaled. Repeat this for 10 breaths.

Herbs are also very effective detoxification—in the form of tea they can be used to ward off a cold or to decrease the severity and length of a cold. The Immune Tonic Tea and Echinacea Lemon Ginger Tea™ given earlier in this chapter are made of herbs that are both cleansing (decreasing the body's burden) and immune system supportive (nourishing and strengthening the self healing mechanism).

Hydrotherapy

HEATING COMPRESS

Heating compresses are wonderfully soothing treatments for colds with and without sore throats. Applying a heating compress differs from a hot compress, which is an application of heat to the body such as soaking gauze in a hot herbal infusion and sponging it on or wrapping it around an injured area of the body. A heating compress is an application of cold that stimulates the body to generate heat. The gift of a heating compress is that it is not doing the work for the body, but stimulating the body's own healing mechanisms into action. Some of the results of a heating compress are an increase in circulation, the elimination of wastes, and the stimulation of the immune system, thus their usefulness in preventing and treating colds.

The Warming Sock Treatment (outlined in Chapter 3) is a heating compress—it gently stimulates circulation, reducing the congestion of a stuffy nose, relieving a sore throat, and loosening up congestion in the lungs from bronchitis as it relieves pain and stimulates the immune response. In addition, it has a sedative effect, facilitating a good night's sleep.

Sore Throat Compress

Another variation of the heating compress useful for a sore throat is the throat compress. This can be done with simple materials from around the house.

MATERIALS

Thin cotton cloth, such as a bandana
Cold water
Essential oil
Wool scarf or piece of wool flannel

INSTRUCTIONS

Soak the cotton cloth completely in cold water. Sprinkle with a few drops of essential oil and wring it out thoroughly so it does not drip.

Warm the neck area with a warm washcloth or by taking a warm shower.

Wrap the cotton cloth around the throat, and then cover it with the wool scarf or cloth. Secure this by tucking in the end of the wool scarf. Leave it on overnight. Your body will quickly generate heat to warm up your throat. The cotton cloth will be dry in the morning.

DOSE / TIMING / DURATION

The throat compress can be used for the duration of a sore throat due to an acute upper respiratory infection. It is safe, and supportive, and can be use nightly.

BENEFITS

This treatment decreases congestion in the throat and head. It is pain relieving and, as with all heating compresses, stimulates the immune response, making it ideal for acute infections. The throat compress has a sedating action that can help you slip into a restful sleep.

INDICATIONS

Sore throat, hoarseness, stiff or painful neck, or any inflammation or infection of the throat.

CAUTIONS

Be careful not to become chilled during the treatment. Keep well covered, and rub your neck briskly if chilling occurs.

I once prescribed this treatment to a seven-year-old boy for his chronically sore throat. His mother was skeptical when I described the treatment, but said she would give it a try. The next time I saw them, the mother exclaimed that *she* wanted to do a heating compress treatment for herself. Her son had loved his throat compress so much, that even after his chronic sore throats went away he still asked for the treatment at night.

FOOT BATHS

The hot foot bath is another hydrotherapy approach to congestion accompanying a cold that merits attention. The hot foot bath employs two processes at once to decrease congestion: drawing and pushing. Blood tends to move toward heat and away from cold. Thus soaking the feet in hot water will draw congestion away from the head and chest. Cold on the head will push congestion away from the head. The hot foot bath detailed here combines this pulling and pushing to relieve headaches caused by congestion.

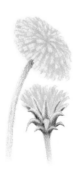

HOT FOOT BATH FOR CONGESTIVE HEADACHES

You will need a tub or large basin of hot water, a wool blanket, 2 washcloths, and a basin with cold water and a few drops of lavender or other essential oil (lavender is particularly good for congestion or headache).

Soak your feet in hot water while wrapped in a warm wool blanket. Make sure the hot footbath remains warm throughout this treatment; move your feet around in the bath and/or add more hot water over time as you can tolerate it. You can have an electrical tea kettle nearby to add hot water as appropriate.

Soak two washcloths in the cold water basin. Place one washcloth on your forehead and relax for 10–15 minutes while you sit comfortably soaking your feet. Alternate with the other cold washcloth frequently so that the one you have on your forehead is always cold.

Take care to avoid getting chilled after this treatment.

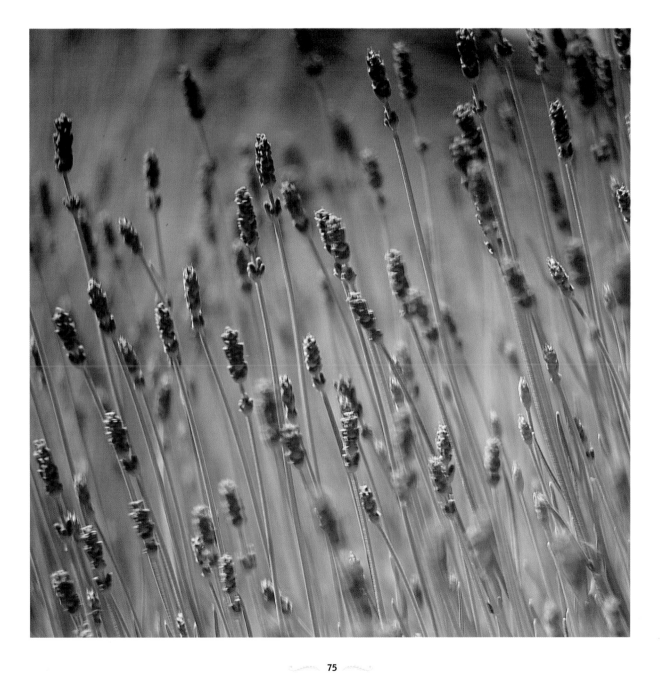

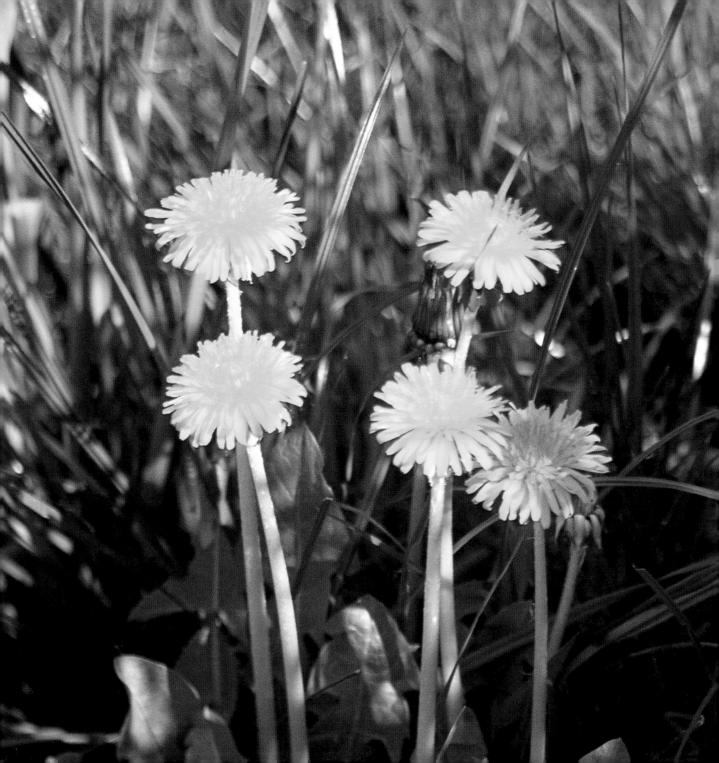

Chapter 6

Hormonal Balance

The scientific understanding of hormonal balance has advanced greatly in the last decade. The wonderful result of this is a much better understanding of many health issues that were previously ignored and left untreated such as depression, pre-menstrual syndrome (PMS), peri-menopause and menopause symptoms, seasonal affectedness disorder, and chronic fatigue. The new information has increased our understanding of hormonal imbalances and presented new opportunities for treating them. Unfortunately, the treatment option that is most often used is direct hormone replacement—that is, if a particular condition is associated with a diminished quantity of a particular hormone, the treatment is to supplement with that hormone. Not only are physicians prescribing hormone replacement more and more frequently, but it is now readily available over the counter. Melatonin, DHEA, progesterone, and estrogen creams are all easily available and being taken after self-diagnosis and prescription.

I think of hormone replacement as a therapy of last resort. Why? The endocrine system is in a constant state of dynamic balance. There are numerous feedback loops, signals from one gland to another, and signals from the brain that cause endocrine glands to produce and secrete hormones. If a given endocrine gland is signaled to either increase or decrease its production because a single hormone is high or low, it not only affects the levels of that particular hormone, but potentially of many others produced or secreted by that same gland. By telling a gland that we need more or less of a given hormone, we are likely to change the production of several other hormones in the body as well—leading to further imbalance.

Hormone supplementation also has the potential for taking over the work of an endocrine gland. If there is sufficient hormone in the bloodstream because it is being supplemented externally, the message to the body is "We don't need to make any more of this hormone." So the body is not stimulated to

produce more and may shut down its own production completely. Once a gland has completely shut down production, it can be extremely difficult to turn it on again.

There are, alternatives to treating directly with hormones, ways that will correct the hormonal imbalance. These include:

- Treating the liver
- Using herbs that nourish and support the endocrine glands
- Using herbs that have hormone-like activity.

Treating the liver plays an important role in correcting hormonal imbalance. Many hormones, including the reproductive hormones—testosterone, estrogens, and progesterone—move through the liver before being excreted. The condition of the liver determines its ability to remove excess hormones from the blood to be excreted via bile into the digestive tract and out of the body. If the liver is congested, overburdened, and overworked, there can be a build up of hormones. A buildup of estrogen, for example, can cause dysmenorrhea, cramping pain, nausea, and vomiting with menstruation. Luckily there are lots of herbs that support the cleansing of the liver—dandelion root, burdock root, red clover, and St. John's wort, just to name a few.

There are also herbs that nourish and support the endocrine glands. Rather than taking over the function of the glands, these herbs provide the glands with specific nutrients, such as B vitamins and much-needed minerals, that are needed to function optimally and can increase activity in a sluggish gland. Some examples of herbs that support adrenal gland functions are Siberian ginseng, gotu kola, avena, and licorice root. Dark green herbs—nettles, cleavers, chickweed, alfalfa, and dandelion—are also nutrient-rich plants that support healthy cell function in every organ of the body. You can easily include these plants in your diet to maintain strong organs and a balanced hormonal system. For example, the dandelions, nettles, and chickweed that grow in your yard can be added to salads or to freshly squeezed carrot or other vegetable juice. To address serious imbalances, larger doses of these plants may be needed.

Using herbs with hormone-like activity is a third way that herbs can be used to support hormonal balance. This is similar to hormone replacement, except that the herbs do not contain the actual hormone—they contain precursors to the hormone. For example, wild yam supports the production of progesterone in the body, vitex berry shows either estrogenic or prog-

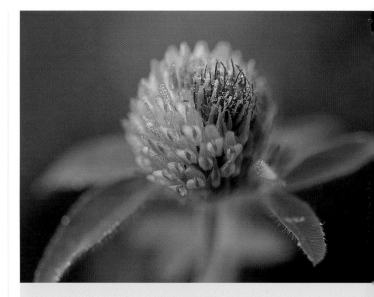

Red clover

esteronic activity, and red clover (the stem and leaf have the most hormone-like activity, whereas the blossom has more liver-cleansing properties) shows slight progesteronic activity. Black cobosh acts as a phyto-estrogen (plant estrogen) and supports women in menopause, influencing hormonal activity related to hot flashes. There is also new research on using herbs for male hormonal imbalances, for example, saw palmetto for prostate health and yohimbe for erectile dysfunction.

HORMONE DISORDERS

Problems with a woman's reproductive cycle can have various causes. It is important to treat the cause—the underlying imbalance—not just the symptoms. There are some herbal treatments such as a cramp bark and kava tea that ease the pain of menstrual cramps. This tea can be a wonderful aid in the treatment of menstrual cramps, it is nontoxic and there is little chance of an adverse reaction. It is, however, only slightly more of a cure than taking aspirin or another pain reliever. The underlying cause is some hormonal imbalance that is causing the menstrual cramps; this is what should be addressed. And, because addressing the underlying problem takes time, and will not give instant relief, a tea such as Menstrual Relief Tea can be used in the meantime to relieve the discomfort.

Fibrocystic breast disease can be effectively treated with the oil from the flower of the evening primrose. This is an example, however, in which the use of herbal therapy alone, as the only treatment, may be disappointing. The most effective treatment for fibrocystic breast disease is the removal of methylxanthines from your diet. These are found in coffee, cola, tea, and chocolate. This is not a situation in which merely decreasing the consumption of these substances will suffice; a complete elimination of them is required to successfully reverse the disease process.

Issues related to women's reproductive cycles—PMS, peri-menopause, menopause, and pregnancy—can all be addressed with the herbs included in the recipes offered here.

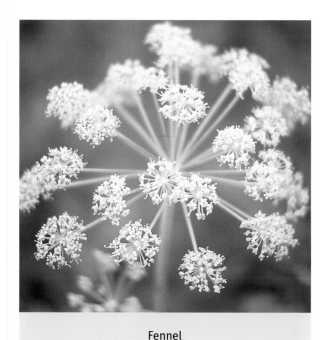

Fennel

Menstrual Relief Tea

INGREDIENTS

  1 part Kava kava
  1 part Cramp bark
  1 part Fennel
  1 part Licorice, orange peel and/or cinnamon
      for flavor

INSTRUCTIONS

Place pure cool water in a sauce pan and add 1 tablespoon of the herb mixture for every cup of water. Bring to a rolling boil. Allow the herbs to simmer for 10 minutes. Turn off the heat and let sit for another 5 minutes. Strain out the herbs and drink the remaining liquid.

DOSE / TIMING / DURATION

On the first day of mesnses, or the day you experience the most discomfort, drink throughout the day as needed, but do not exceed 8 cups. If you drink this tea for more than 1 day, an appropriate dose would be 1–4 cups per day.

BENEFITS

Relieves muscle cramping and spasm specifically of the uterus, urinary, and intestinal tracts. The herbs in this tea are pain relieving and anti-inflammatory. Kava, specifically, relieves muscle spasms and anxiety. It is calming, but does not diminish cognitive function like most sedatives.

INDICATIONS

I have placed this tea here as a treatment for menstrual cramps. It is very effective in this, and it is also useful for other conditions involving muscle spasm, such as tension headaches, urinary tract spasm, and intestinal cramping.

CAUTIONS

- Kava kava should not be used during pregnancy or while nursing. It can enhance the sleep-inducing effects of alcohol. Caution should be used in the operation of heavy machinery or when driving while using kava because muscle coordination may be diminished.

- Kava kava can cause a skin rash (dry, pigmented, and scaly) when used in large doses for extended periods of time. The rash will resolve once you stop taking it.

- Kava kava should not be used with other medications or with alcohol. See Chapter 2 for a discussion of the safety of kava kava.

- Cramp bark should not be used with blood-thinning medications because it contains coumarin. Although cramp bark is used therapeutically during pregnancy, it should only be used in this circumstance with the supervision of a health-care professional.

Women's Balance Tea™

INGREDIENTS

1/4 part Vitex berry
1 part St. John's wort buds
1 part Motherwort herb
1 part Dandelion leaf
1 part Peppermint leaf

INSTRUCTIONS

Using your favorite tea-making tool (tea pot, French press, infusing basket, or tea ball), add a heaping teaspoon of the herb mixture for each cup of just boiled water. Cover and let sit for approximately 5 minutes. Pour the tea into a cup, straining out the herbs (or remove the infusing basket or tea ball), inhale the tea's aroma, and sip slowly.

DOSE / TIMING / DURATION

Drink 1–4 cups per day; 3 or 4 cups per day is considered a therapeutic dosage. Such a dosage could be taken for 3 weeks and discontinued the week of menstruation. Continue 3 weeks on and 1 week off for at least 3 months to see long-term changes in hormonal balance. A single cup of this tea anytime can be soothing, calming, and nutritious.

BENEFITS

Re-establishing balance between estrogen and progesterone, cleansing via the liver and the kidneys, and tonifying to the heart. It is also a diuretic, bringing relief to bloating due to hormonal fluctuation.

INDICATIONS

This tea is designed to bring relief of the many symptoms that women experience due to hormonal fluctuation and imbalance. These include premenstrual and peri-menopausal symptoms such as bloating and weight gain, depression, anxiety and irritability, vaginal dryness, hot flashes, and insomnia.

CAUTIONS

Caution should be used in taking St. John's wort with anti-depressant medications, anti-HIV drugs, and birth control pills and also around surgery.

Nutritive Vinegar for Women

INGREDIENTS

1 part Dandelion leaf
1 part Red raspberry leaf
Apple cider vinegar

INSTRUCTIONS

Place the fresh or dried herbs into a jar, cover with apple cider vinegar and fasten with a nonmetal lid. Let the mixture cure for 6 weeks. Strain out the herbs by pouring the vinegar through cheesecloth, and squeeze the herbs in the cheesecloth tightly. The vinegar can be stored in a bottle at room temperature.

If desired red raspberry leaf can be combined with other green leaves to provide a deeply nourishing tea with protein, vitamins, and minerals and also a mild diuretic action. Herbs to consider include dandelion leaf, alfalfa, and nettles.

DOSE / TIMING / DURATION

Take 1 tablespoon up to 3 times daily in a cup of water.

BENEFITS

This tonic is supportive of digestion and assimilation of nutrients. Diuretic effects relieve bloating associated with hormonal fluctuation. Red raspberry leaf improves uterine tone, strengthens the uterus, eases childbirth, promotes the flow of breast milk, prevents miscarriage, and strengthens vasculature.

INDICATIONS

This is a wonderful tonic for pregnancy. Also useful for heavy and painful menses, edema, and varicose veins. This tonic is generally supportive of hormonal balance in women in their child-bearing years.

CAUTIONS

Dandelion should not be used in acute conditions of the gallbladder or intestinal tract.

Red Raspberry Leaf Tea

INGREDIENTS

Red raspberry leaf

INSTRUCTIONS

Using your favorite tea-making tool (tea pot, French press, infusing basket, or tea ball), add a heaping teaspoon of the herb to each cup of just boiled water. Cover and let sit for approximately 5 minutes. Pour the tea into a cup, straining out the herbs (or remove the infusing basket or tea ball), inhale the tea's aroma, and sip slowly.

DOSE / TIMING / DURATION

Drink 2–3 cups per day.

BENEFITS

Helps to regulate hormonal balance and is calming, soothing, and gently relaxing without making you drowsy. It helps build up nervous system tissue, providing strength and endurance. It is especially appropriate for pregnancy because it strengthens the muscles of the uterus, preventing miscarriages and easing childbirth; it also promotes the flow of breast milk.

INDICATIONS

Pregnancy and lactation, nervous irritability and fatigue, PMS, or menstrual discomfort. A perfect tea for expectant mothers or worn-out new mothers.

CAUTIONS

The use of red raspberry leaf may not be indicated where there is a history of sudden labor. In such a situation, it is best to use the herb under the supervision of a healthcare practitioner familiar with the use of herbs.

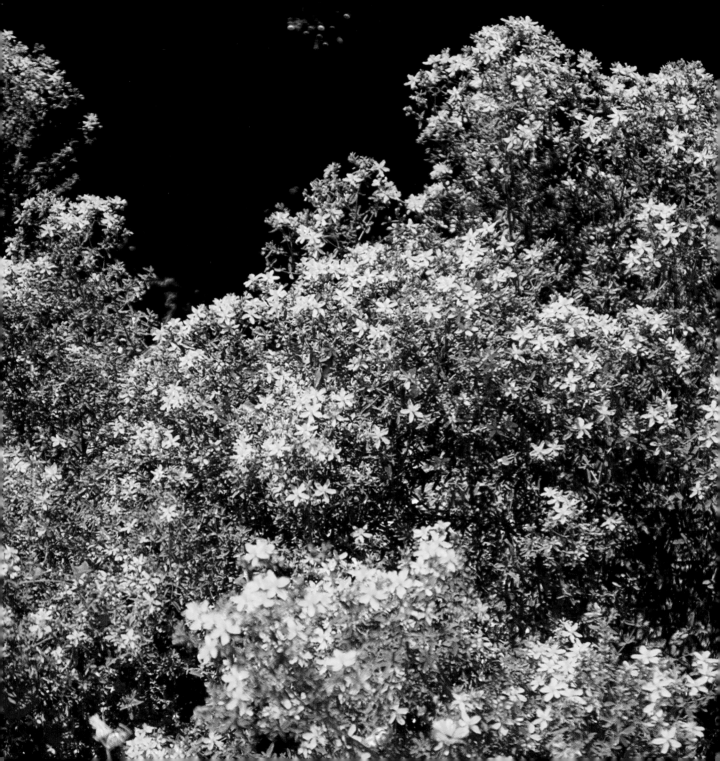

Chapter 7

Emotional Balance

Managing our moods and emotions has become a big point of focus lately. Prescriptions for Prozac and other antidepressant drugs seem to be given out like candy. And in the case of the natural pharmacy; once it became known that the herb St. John's wort could successfully treat mild to moderate depression, its sales skyrocketed.

There is a tendency in American culture to think that our emotions should be consistent. We always want to feel happy and full of energy. When we do not, we think something is wrong. Actually the life within us has the capacity for a great number of emotional experiences, and these are all a part of life. Joy, sadness, anger, grieving, and loneliness are some of the many emotions we might

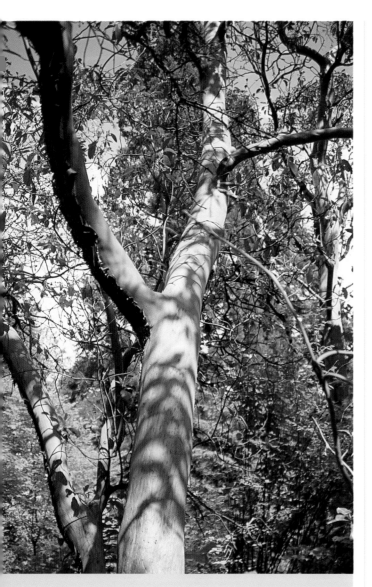

Madrone

experience. These emotions can all be appropriate responses to life, just as many different levels of energy are appropriate at different times of the day, week, and month and over the course of a life. We have a tendency to expect a consistent face from ourselves and from those around us, and if that is not the case we ask, "What is wrong?"

This is another area where we can learn by observing the plants around us. Trees drop their leaves in the fall and go into a quiet, less expressive state in the winter. In the spring they burst forth with flowers and fresh green leaves, and then in the summer they bear fruit. For trees, spring and summer are times of great expression, extroversion, and exchange with its environment, whereas winter seems to be a time of introversion, taking their energy inside and building it so that in the spring they will be able to begin producing outwardly again. In the wintertime, do trees feel deficient? Do they think that they are ill because they do not have flowers or that nobody will like them because they aren't producing shade or fruit? Of course not, trees are totally content with their state in each season. Cycles of change are a natural part of life, and really no state is better than any other. And as trees show us, one state can be crucial for the existence of another state at another time.

Thus as we move through life we will feel sad, happy, courageous, fearful, angry, irritable, anxious, calm, relaxed, and agitated—and there is no problem with any of these states. Each one can be an appropriate response at a particular moment. Problems develop when we get stuck in one of these states and we can't get out. An emotional state becomes pathological when it takes over and controls us. And our desire to have a consistent emotional state can lead to imbalance—a one-sided emotional picture—which does not represent health.

If you don't feel like smiling or don't feel particularly happy, then you may begin to think that something is wrong with you. Why can't you be happy all the time? So perhaps you begin to do things in excess that have made you happy in the past, such as drinking alcohol or taking in a large amount of caffeine or sugar. These activities, although they may make you feel happy in the short run, in the long run create an imbalance in the body and become depressants. This kind of cycle can take a normal everyday emotion, a moment of melancholy, and turn it into a pathological state, true depression.

The first step in the use of herbs to keep us emotionally balanced is using them to ease our way through the day-to-day ups and downs. These tools are unlikely to provide a complete cure when an emotional state has become extreme, but in the early stages, when we are first thrown off-balance, they can be used to simply restore balance. When the condition has become extreme, these same tools can be used as part of a fuller program for restoring balance.

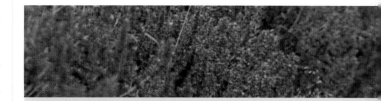

LAVENDER RELAXING BATH

On a busy and stressful day, we might choose to take a lavender bath to release muscle tension and calm our agitated mental state.

Place a handful of lavender buds in a piece of cheesecloth, muslin, or a thin sock. Tie a string around the top to close the opening or, if you are using a sock, tie the top in a knot. Place this bundle of herbs under the faucet as you fill the bathtub. Hot water will best extract the healing properties of the plant, so use water as hot as you can make it to fill the bath, and then let it cool to a comfortable temperature before immersing yourself into the herbal bath. (For other herbs to use in a relaxing bath, see the recipe for Calming Herbal Baths in Chapter 11.)

Holistic Approaches to Depression

The other way to use herbs for emotional balance is to treat the imbalance after it has occurred. In holistic health modalities, we always strive to treat the cause and not just the symptoms. The answer, therefore, to a depressed mood is not simply to artificially elevate the mood but to find out what has caused the prolonged depression in the first place. Many of the true causes of depression are well addressed with herbs.

LIVER CONGESTION

One common cause of depression is liver congestion. This can occur via the scenario already described—a slight imbalance in mood leads us to use a substance that temporarily lifts our spirits, such as an antidepressant medication, alcohol, coffee, or cigarettes, but then leaves the body with a toxic burden that it must get rid of. This puts strain on the liver, which functions to keep the blood flowing to every cell in our body full of nutrients that support cell function and clear of toxins that inhibit cell function (see Chapter 4 for a discussion of liver function).

When the liver is overburdened, it can become congested and unable to do many of its functions: blood purification, production of crucial digestive substances, and the production of energy in the body. The liver performs so many complex and vital functions in the body it is no wonder that naturopathic physicians treat the liver to cure an enormous variety of ailments.

Liver congestion is treated very effectively with herbs. Herbs such as dandelion root, burdock root, and St. John's wort buds are some of the many herbs that purify the blood through their action on the liver. Both dandelion and burdock roots are tonifying herbs that can be taken over long periods of time. In fact, they are very effectively used as a regular part of our diet to promote wellness, not just as medicine after an imbalance has set in. Dandelion and burdock roots can be made into a tea. Because they are roots, they should be decocted (boiled; see Chapter 13 for a description of decoctions) to most effectively extract the healing properties of the herbs. Here is a sample recipe of a liver cleansing tea.

Liver Cleansing Tea

INGREDIENTS

1 part Burdock root
1 part Dandelion root
1/4 part Licorice root, fennel seeds, or orange peel (for flavoring)

INSTRUCTIONS

Place pure cool water in a sauce pan and add 1 tablespoon of the herb mixture for every cup of water. Bring to a rolling boil. Allow the herbs to simmer for 10 minutes. Turn off the heat and let sit for another 5 minutes. Strain out the herbs and drink the remaining liquid.

DOSE / TIMING / DURATION

Drink 3–4 cups per day. These herbs are tonics to the body and can be used safely on an ongoing basis.

BENEFITS

Detoxifies, promotes digestion and absorption of nutrients, decreases inflammation, supports elimination through the digestive tract, and protects the liver from toxic substances.

INDICATIONS

Depression, PMS, and other problems with hormonal shifts, acne, eczema, and muscle and joint pain.

CAUTIONS

- Licorice root increases sodium reabsorption, causing water retention. High doses are therefore contraindicated in cases of hypertension, congestive heart failure, and kidney disease. Doses of 3 grams (approximately 1 tablespoon) or more of licorice root a day should not be taken for more than 6 weeks, unless monitored by a healthcare practitioner.

- Oregon grape root should not be used during pregnancy because it contains several compounds that stimulate the uterus.

- Remember that it is a good idea to take a break from any herb that you use regularly. Take a 2-week break every 3–4 months, or rotate your herbs every few months. In the case of the liver cleansing herbs, consider rotating from the list given here, changing the combination for 3–4 months, and then changing it again, continuing in this manner for as long as desired or indicated.

Dandelion root
Burdock root
Yellow dock root
Milk thistle seed
Oregon grape root
Licorice root

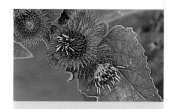

Burdock

Emotional Health and Brain Function

Another way that we can use herbs to support emotional balance is to look at the role of hormones and neurotransmitters on brain function. Modern science has developed antidepressant drugs that act on neurotransmitters in the brain as a method of controlling emotions. These medications inhibit mono-amine oxidase (MAO inhibitors) and the re-uptake of serotonin (SSRIs). St. John's wort is an herbal alternative.

ST. JOHN'S WORT

While I was still a Naturopathic medical student—early in my botanical training—I remember walking with one of my professors, Dr. Jill Stansbury, a very fine herbalist/botanist and master of plants and their chemical constituents, and mentioning with surprise that hypericum (St. John's wort) had just appeared in my garden that year. It hadn't been there the previous year, and then suddenly it was popping up all over! Jill smiled and said, "That's because you're an herbalist. The plants find you." At

the time, I definitely did not think that I qualified for the title of herbalist, but it made me happy to hear her say it, and maybe her saying it actually made it so.

I can't tell you how many times I have shown the St. John's wort in my garden to my friends with excitement and gotten the response, "That's St. Johns wort? It looks like a weed!!!" It's true that St. John's wort has a very unassuming presence. It has a tall, thin stem branching outward at an unglamorous angle and leading to very small yellow flowers. The flowers are beautiful up close, but from a distance the plant has the appearance of a spindly roadside weed.

In Oregon, where I live, St. John's wort does grow like a weed. It has a reputation for taking over open fields. It can be a nuisance for livestock raisers—cows grazing on fields of St. John's wort can develop an increased sensitivity to sunlight and become severely burned. The herb can also be a nuisance for gardeners because its seeds spread quickly and easily, and, once it has taken root, it takes some work to dig it out. But the label *weed* is all in the eye of the beholder—some of the plants that we call weeds are the most nourishing plants on the planet. They grow easily and in abundance and spread themselves from one location to another to make themselves easily accessible to as many people as possible. What a gift!

That first year St. John's wort appeared in my garden, I was so thrilled I dug it up from the pathways and transplanted it into my garden beds.

St. John's wort has been studied as a natural alternative to the common antidepressant drugs. Originally, it was thought to act by one of the same mechanisms as the MAO inhibitors and SSRIs. As scientific studies on St. John's wort continued, it became apparent that its mechanism was neither of these. Herbalists have been aware for a long time that St. John's wort acts on the liver, which purifies the blood. This may very well be the mechanism by which it alleviates depression.

In studying St. John's wort, scientists focused on its constituent hypericin to try to understand its antidepressant effects. Companies that make standardized extracts began standardizing the hypericin content of their St. John's wort preparations. After further research, scientists found that hypericin was not responsible for the antidepressant effects of St. John's wort after all; instead hyperfolin—another constituent of the plant—was responsible. Extracts were then standardized to that constituent. It is highly possible that neither one of these constituents alone is responsible for the antidepressant effects of St. John's wort but that the entire medley of plant constituents found in the plant acts synergistically

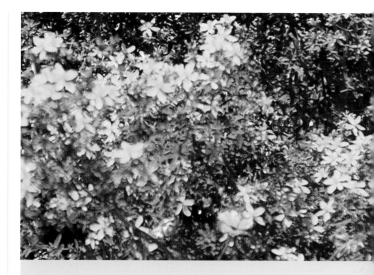

St. John's wort

to have the multitude of effects of St. John's wort. My inclination is that we should leave the wisdom of nature alone and adulterate the herb as little as possible.

Tea brings the herb to us in its whole form, allowing us to benefit from its mood-balancing properties without having to know its true mechanism or active ingredient. In herbal mythology, St. John's wort and calendula (also featured in the tea that follows) are associated with the sun, letting light into dark places. The following recipe is warming and uplifting—just what's needed on a gray day.

Cup of Sunshine Tea™

INGREDIENTS

1-1/2 parts Ginkgo biloba
1-1/2 parts St. John's wort
1/2 part Red clover
1 part Calendula
1/4 part Ginger
1 part Lemon grass

INSTRUCTIONS

Using your favorite tea-making tool (tea pot, French press, infusing basket, or tea ball) add 1 heaping teaspoon of the herb mixture to each cup of just boiled water. Cover and let sit for approximately 5 minutes. Pour the tea into a cup, straining out the herbs (or remove the infusing basket or tea ball), inhale the tea's aroma, and sip slowly.

DOSE / TIMING / DURATION

Drink 1–4 cups per day; 3 or 4 cups per day is considered a therapeutic dosage. This dosage should be used for at least 3 weeks, and up to 3 months, to achieve the long-term benefits of these herbs. However, a single cup anytime can be invigorating in the short term.

BENEFITS

This tea is one of the recipes I formulated for my company The Art of Health, Inc. It contains herbs that support emotional balance from many perspectives. St. John's wort and red clover blossoms are both liver cleansers; ginkgo supports blood flow to the brain and throughout the body, helping to deliver vital nutrients to cells; and ginger and calendula relieve stagnation of blood and lymph.

INDICATIONS

Mild to moderate depression, depression associated with menopause, and depression in the elderly.

CAUTIONS

- St. John's wort (hypericum) should be used with caution when taking antidepressant medications. Consult with a healthcare professional knowledgeable in the use of herbs and familiar with the potential drug interactions. Having a knowledgeable healthcare professional monitor your use of both the herb and the medications, as well as your progress and response, is most likely to lead to successful treatment without adverse reactions.

- St. John's wort may cause skin hypersensitivity to sunlight.

- Ginkgo and St. John's wort should not be taken directly before or after surgery.

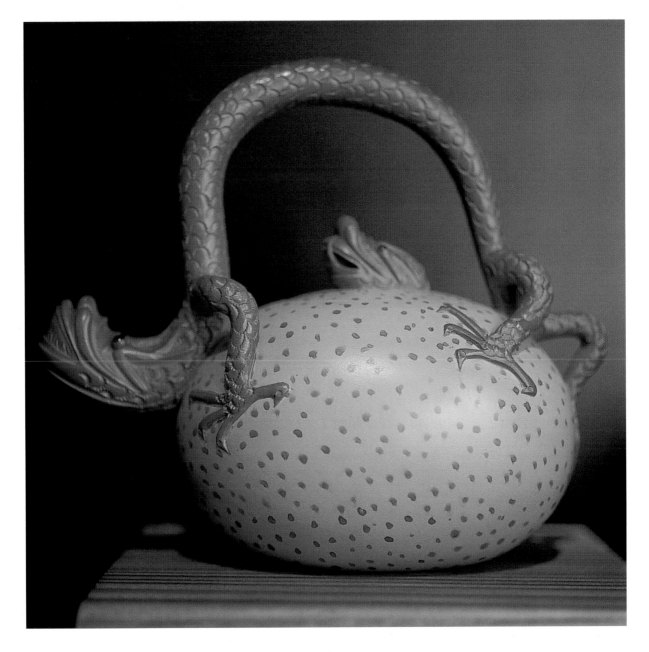

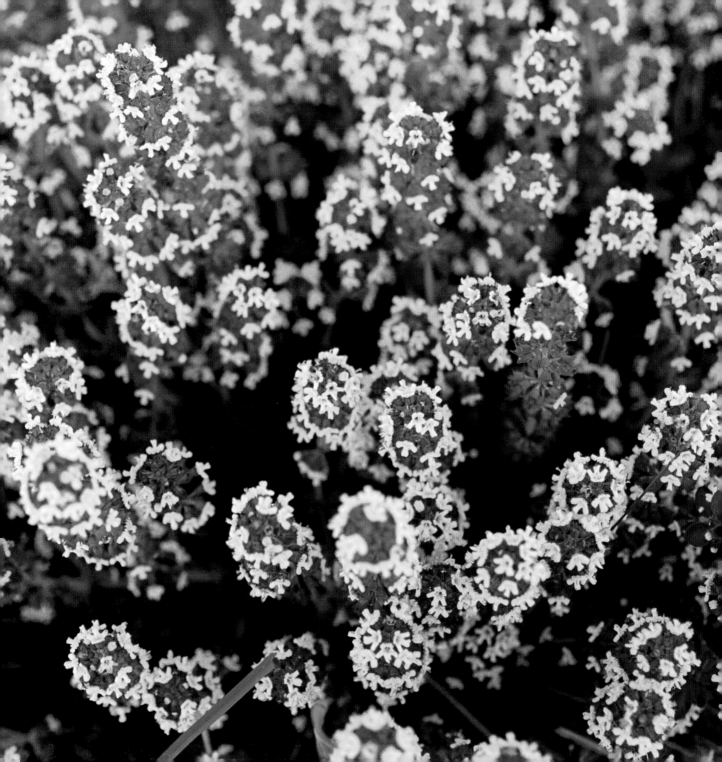

Chapter 8

Breathing Freely

The respiratory tract is one of the body's important mechanisms for exchange with our environment. It is through the respiratory tract that we take in the oxygen needed by every cell in the body to function and eliminate carbon dioxide, the most abundant waste product in the body. Effective respiration is crucial to maintain life. As with the heart (see Chapter 9), the disruption of the free flow of this system can be life threatening, causing, for example, an acute asthma attack. And, as with the digestive tract (see Chapter 4), there can be a lower-grade dysfunction of this system for which the body compensates over relatively long periods of time until it finally becomes overwhelmed and the symptoms of illness appear. If we ignore these low-grade symptoms, treating them as minor annoyances, we find that down the road we have serious symptoms that are very disruptive to our well-being and are more difficult to treat.

A Healthy Respiratory Tract

The respiratory tract is elegantly designed to make this gas exchange, this interaction with our external environment, happen efficiently. Air contains many other particles in it other than oxygen, such as dust, molds, and pollutants. These can harm the body if they are inhaled into the lungs, so the respiratory tract is armed with tools to filter out unwanted particles as it draws air into the body. The nose is armed with hairs that catch dust particles in the inhaled air, keeping them from entering the trachea. The nose is also designed so that the air is swirled around a large surface area, which warms and mois-

Most of us generally breathe quite shallowly. This is a response to stress and the build up of tension that occurs when we are unable to respond fully and appropriately to stressful situations. This is yet another example of how stress affects the function of every system in the body.

tens the air so that by the time the air moves further into the respiratory tract and contacts the more delicate internal structures it is body temperature. The tract itself is lined with cilia. These are tiny fibers along the walls that brush particles up and out of the respiratory tract keeping them from settling in the lungs. Finally, deep in the lung tissue there are immune system cells—macrophages that swallow up particles that have made it past the cilia.

MAINTAINING A HEALTHY RESPIRATORY TRACT

Most problems of the upper and lower respiratory tract are preventable. Air quality is key. Avoiding polluted air and not smoking are important, of course. But because air pollution is increasingly pervasive and difficult to avoid, we need to do whatever we can to enhance lung function. Go for walks in heavily wooded areas. Breathe deeply to cleanse the respiratory tract. Through exercising or deep breathing through yoga, you increase the rate and volume of exhaled air. These are important tools you can employ to enhance this natural detoxifying body function. Herbs can also enhance lung function by facilitating detoxification and tonifying respiratory tissues.

Lung Cleansing Tea

If you are chronically exposed to polluted air in your home or work environment, or have residual lung congestion after an infection, the Lung Cleansing Tea offered here helps clear the lungs and restore healthy function.

INGREDIENTS

1 part Fenugreek seeds
1/4 part Ginger root (or to taste)
1 part Fennel seeds
1/4 part Licorice root (or to taste)

INSTRUCTIONS

Place pure cool water in a sauce pan and add 1 tablespoon of the herb mixture for every cup of water. Bring to a rolling boil. Allow the herbs to simmer for 10 minutes. Turn off the heat and let sit for another 5 minutes. Strain out the herbs, breathe the warm steam in through your nose deeply into your lungs, and drink.

DOSE / TIMING / DURATION

Drink 3–4 cups per day. This tea can be used daily for extended periods of time.

BENEFITS

Disperses cold and reduces inflammation. Mildly expectorating and antispasmodic. Mucilaginous properties soothe and heal irritated respiratory passageways.

INDICATIONS

This is a nice-tasting tea that can be used every day over an extended period of time to cleanse and support the lungs. It is useful for that lingering cough after a difficult winter of bronchitis or pneumonia. It is a nice tea to use as a follow-up after a bad cough for which you were taking strong herbs like osha. When you are mostly recovered and the taste of osha becomes too much, this tea makes a nice transition. Milder in taste and fragrance, it keeps the attention on the lungs, on expectorating any lingering residue and supporting healthy function.

CAUTIONS

Fenugreek should not be used during pregnancy due to its potential to stimulate the onset of menses and cause abortion.

Treating Impaired Respiratory Function

What should we do when we are not able to breathe freely, when our respiratory tract is not functioning optimally? There are some simple ways that you can use herbs to facilitate easier breathing. Some of these bring symptomatic relief. If the illness is short-lived, such as a stuffy, congested head cold, symptomatic treatment may be the only treatment that the respiratory tract needs. Once the cold is over, free breathing will be restored naturally.

There are many situations, however, where a more systemic treatment approach is needed. If the respiratory restriction is due to allergies, for instance, the allergies themselves need to be addressed. Herbs may be an important part of this treatment as well. If there has been some chronic irritation to the respiratory tract that over time has led to diminished function—smoking, for example, causes this kind of damage—the treatment approach must include a removal of the cause, in this case smoking cigarettes, as well as some specific support to heal and regenerate the damaged tissues. The latter is when herbs again play a role.

CLEARING CONGESTION

Congestion of the upper respiratory tract may be due to head colds or allergies. For symptoms of the upper respiratory tract such as stuffy nose, itchy eyes, and clogged sinuses herbs can be used to decrease congestion, open the passageways, and relieve itching and lacrimation from nose, eyes, and throat. The herbs in my Allergy Clearing Detox Tea™ are specific for symptoms caused by hay fever or other allergic response, but they also work beautifully if the symptoms are due to a head cold. In this case, you might consider adding echinacea flowering tops to boost the immune system while addressing the congestion in the head.

Hydrotherapy can also be highly effective in treating congestion of the upper respiratory tract. For example, you can use the steam inhalation described in the next section, or you can apply the warming sock treatment (described in Chapter 3) to help keep the nasal passageways open at night so you can sleep.

Allergy Clearing Detox Tea™

INGREDIENTS

Eyebright
Nettles
Licorice root
Rose hips
Red clover

Use equal parts of each herb.

INSTRUCTIONS

Using your favorite tea-making tool (tea pot, French press, infusing basket, or tea ball), add 1 heaping teaspoon of the herb mixture for each cup of just boiled water. Cover and let sit for approximately 5 minutes. Pour the tea into a cup, straining out the herbs (or remove the infusing basket or tea ball), inhale the tea's aroma, and sip slowly.

DOSE/TIMING/DURATION

One cup can be taken at any time to bring almost instant relief to symptoms of allergies; 3–4 cups daily can be taken on an ongoing basis to support detoxification and decrease the body's reactivity to potential allergens.

BENEFITS

Nettles and red clover cleanse the body of excessive toxic burden through action on the liver and kidneys. The anti-inflammatory properties of licorice, eyebright, and rose hips contribute to the tea's ability to calm the inflammation and excessive discharges of the nasal passages and respiratory tract associated with allergies.

INDICATIONS

Hayfever, eczema, and other allergies, and as an aid in detoxification.

CAUTIONS

- Very large quantities of nettles should be avoided during pregnancy due to its potential to bring on menses. It is, however, recommended for pregnant women in small amounts for its nutritive properties.

- Regular use of red clover is also contra-indicated during pregnancy.

- Red clover increases the action of blood-thinning medications. If you are on these medications and consuming red clover, have your blood viscosity monitored regularly.

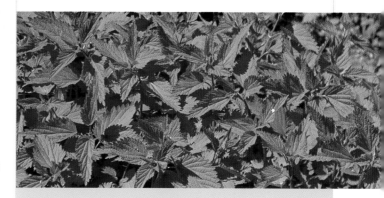

Nettles

RELEASING SPASM

There is a group of herbs called antispasmodics. These can be used to relieve a tight constrictive cough or when there is loss of elasticity in the tissue, bronchoconstriction, inflammation, and spasm of the respiratory passageways, which occur in the chronic obstructive pulmonary diseases (COPD)—chronic bronchitis, asthma, and emphysema.

Asthma is a very common obstructive lung disease. When acute, it is serious and can lead to death. Treatment of an acute asthma attack should always be under the supervision of a qualified healthcare professional. Chronic asthma can be treated effectively with herbs, but it is important that the treatment be focused on the cause. Asthma can be allergic—caused by an allergy to substances such as pollen, food, mold, animals, or drugs; or it can be nonallergic—caused by a respiratory tract infection, irritants, or emotional factors; or it can be caused by a combination of these. In each case, it is important to treat the cause, not just the asthmatic symptoms.

Antispasmodic herbs relieve constriction, decrease inflammation, and reduce the narrowing of the passageways and excessively thick secretions. They can be taken internally as a tea, in capsules, or as a tincture, or they can be taken externally via steam inhalation.

DEEP LUNG CLEANSING— GETTING THE GUNK OUT

For infectious diseases of the lungs, you can use mucilaginous herbs to help thin excessively thick secretions, expectorating herbs to remove the mucus from the lungs, and immune-stimulating and antimicrobial herbs to support the body conquer the invading pathogen. These herbs can be taken as teas or through the Herbal Steam Inhalation for Sinuses and Lungs. The bath and sweat recipe given next provides an external use of hydrotherapy and herbs to loosen thickened mucus and facilitate deep lung cleansing.

Pneumonia is an example of a lower respiratory tract infection that should respond well to these therapies: hot drinks, herbal inhalations, and the bath and sweat treatment. Pneumonia should resolve in 1 week; if it doesn't respond quickly to home therapies, it is important to consult a healthcare provider.

Herbs that decrease inflammation are useful in almost every respiratory formula. Licorice root and rose hips are included in the Allergy Clearing Detox Tea™ on page 99 for their anti-inflammatory properties.

Herbal Steam Inhalation for Sinuses and Lungs

INGREDIENTS

1/2 cup dried herb or 5–10 drops of the essential oil of one of the herbs in Table 3 on page 103.

INSTRUCTIONS

Place a small sauce pan on the stove and add 3 cups of water. Heat until steaming. Turn off the heat. To keep from burning yourself on the hot pan, you can pour the steaming hot water into a ceramic bowl, which either contains your dried herbs or to which you add 5–10 drops of the essential oil.

For the Sinuses
Place your head in the path of the steam and breathe in deeply through the nose and then breathe out through the nose. Breathe in again through the mouth and out through the mouth. Breathe in through the nose again and breathe out through the nose. Take a break; then repeat two more times. If one nasal passageway is more congested than the other, breathe in through the open nostril then close this nostril by pressing your hand against it and breathe out through the congested nostril. Repeat this several times.

For the Lungs
Breathe in deeply through the mouth and then out through the mouth. Then breathe in through the nose and out through the nose. Again, breathe in through the mouth and out through the mouth. Take a break; then repeat two more times.

DOSE / TIMING / DURATION

The process may be repeated three times throughout the day. It is important not to take more than the three breaths, as described in the instructions, at any one time because the essential oils can become irritants to the mucus membranes of the respiratory tract.

BENEFITS AND INDICATIONS

See Table 3 on page 103.

CAUTIONS

- Do not use a towel or other object over the head as a tent because this can lead to the burning of the face or respiratory passageways.

- See Table 3 on page 103.

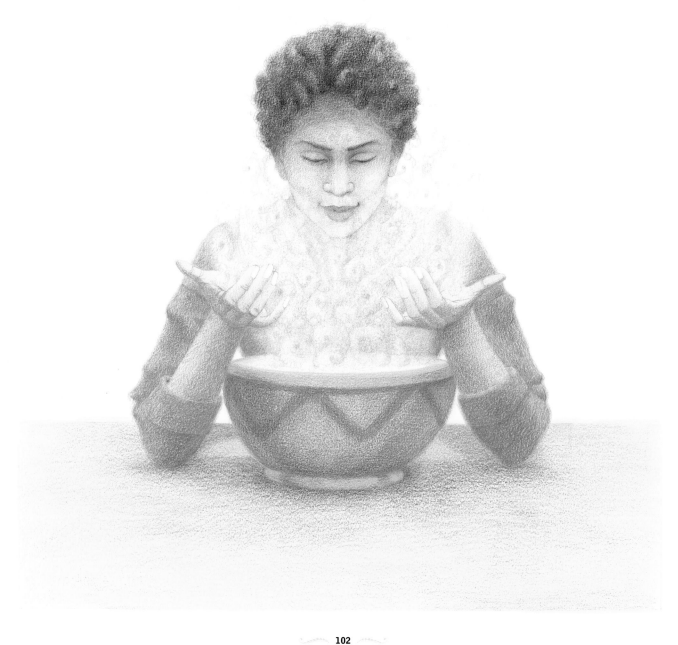

Table 3 Herbs for Steam Inhalation

HERBS	BENEFITS	INDICATIONS	CAUTIONS
Eucalyptus	Clears sinus congestion, is expectorating, destroys bacteria	Head cold with nasal and sinus congestion	No contraindications for external use
Chamomile	Is antispasmodic, destroys bacteria	Tight or spastic cough, asthma, bronchitis	No contraindications for external use
Thyme	Is expectorating, destroys bacteria	Congestion in the lungs accompanying a cold or flu	May cause irritation or allergic reaction in sensitive individuals

Table 4 Types of Respiratory Herbs

Antispasmodic herbs	Garlic, osha, chamomile, peppermint, wild cherry bark, red clover, thyme, valerian, and mullein
Mucilaginous herbs	Althea, garlic and onions, licorice, wild cherry bark, comfrey, slippery elm, and mullein
Expectorating herbs	Eucalyptus, osha root, ginger, and mullein (with resin) Cherry bark and mullein (relaxing)
Anti-microbial herbs	Garlic, onion, Oregon grape, calendula, echinacea, angustifolia, osha, and thyme
Anti-inflammatory herbs	Licorice root, rose hips

Bath and Sweat Treatment

MATERIALS

1/2 cup dried Ginger root or 2 inches of fresh ginger
root, thinly sliced
Cotton sock or piece of gauze
Bathtub
Small basin full of ice water
Washcloth or ice pack
Glass of ice water for drinking
Warm clothing

INSTRUCTIONS

This is a strong treatment. If possible, it is good to have a helper who can set up the bath, perhaps help with the cold friction, make the ginger poultice and so on.

Make a poultice out of ginger. You can do this by placing the ginger in a piece of gauze or in a sock that you knot at the end to make a little bag. Fill the bathtub with hot water, letting the water from the faucet fall onto your ginger compress. Fill a small basin by the side of the bathtub with ice water and place the washcloth in it to soak. Also prepare a glass of ice water for drinking.

Once the bath has cooled to a comfortable temperature, get into the bathtub and soak for 5–10 minutes. During this time, take the ginger compress and dab it over the lungs, resoaking it in the bath periodically. During this time, place the cold washcloth (or an ice pack) over your forehead,

refreshing it as it warms up. Sip the cool water as needed. After 5–10 minutes, stand up and resoak the washcloth in ice water. Wrap the washcloth around your hand and rub it briskly over your chest, arms, and upper back. Add more hot water to the bath if it has cooled, and get back in it for another 5–10 minutes. This process is repeated three times. After the final repetition, step completely out of the bathtub and do the cold friction rub over the entire body, even the feet.

Then go to bed. To intensify the sweating aspect of the treatment, you can get dressed very warmly (i.e., in sweatpants and sweatshirt, socks, gloves, and even a hat and scarf). Get into bet and sweat it out.

DOSE / TIMING / DURATION

Use this treatment once daily during acute illness. Use it when you are settling in for bed for the evening or when the illness keeps you in bed all day. Do *not* expect to get up and do *anything* for several hours after the bath. A treatment as strong as this should not be necessary for more than 3–5 days. If the illness persists in its intensity beyond this time, consult a healthcare practitioner.

BENEFITS

This is a great therapy for times when the whole body aches. It is pain relieving, facilitates

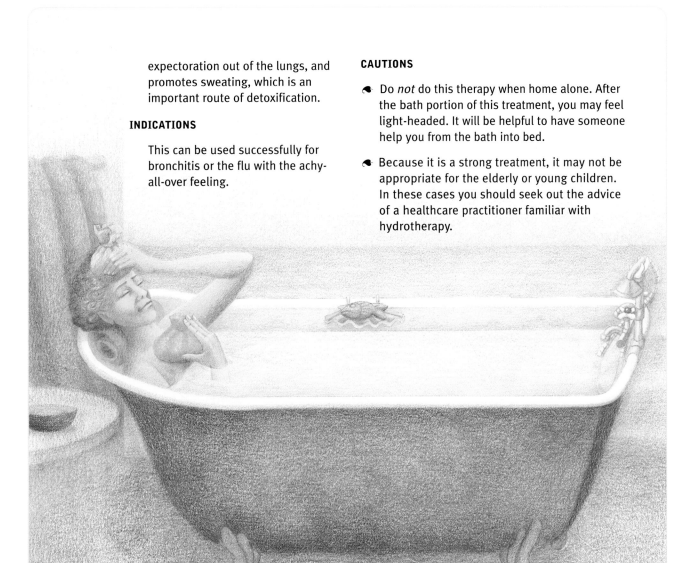

expectoration out of the lungs, and promotes sweating, which is an important route of detoxification.

INDICATIONS

This can be used successfully for bronchitis or the flu with the achy-all-over feeling.

CAUTIONS

● Do *not* do this therapy when home alone. After the bath portion of this treatment, you may feel light-headed. It will be helpful to have someone help you from the bath into bed.

● Because it is a strong treatment, it may not be appropriate for the elderly or young children. In these cases you should seek out the advice of a healthcare practitioner familiar with hydrotherapy.

Mucilaginous Herbs

Mucilaginous herbs are very important in treating respiratory ailments. They soothe inflamed respiratory passageways caused by asthma, bronchitis, and coughs. Mucilage hydrates the mucosal surfaces of the respiratory tract, helping to thin the mucus and make it easier to expectorate. Old accumulations of mucus tend to be thick and difficult to remove.

Expectorating Herbs

The action of expectorating herbs in respiratory infections is obvious. They act by irritating the respiratory passageways. This irritation causes the body to secrete fresh, thin mucus that is easily expectorated.

Expectorating herbs that also contain resins are warming and stimulating, expectorating, and anti-microbial; this makes them especially useful in treating respiratory infections. Because irritation of the tissues causes their expectorating action, they are best used for short periods of time during an acute phase of illness.

There is another group of expectorating herbs that can be called relaxing expectorants. These plants tend to contain mucilage and have antispasmodic properties. They hydrate and relax the respiratory tissues. They are especially useful for tight, dry coughs. These herbs calm bronchial spasms while promoting mucus secretion and thinning thick accumulations in the respiratory passageways.

Anti-Microbial Herbs

Anti-microbial herbs destroy invading viruses or bacteria. The Immune-Boost Cough and Cold Tea provides a good way to take them. A tasty way to getting the anti-microbial properties of garlic and onions is by taking the Cough and Cold Syrup for Children described in Chapter 11.

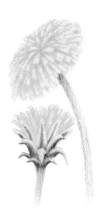

Immune-Boost Cough and Cold Tea

INGREDIENTS

1 part *Echinacea purpurea*
1 part *Echinacea angustifolia*
1/2 part Wild cherry bark
1/2 part Osha root
1/4 part Cinnamon
1/4 part Ginger
1/4 part Cardamom
Honey (optional)

INSTRUCTIONS

Place pure cool water in a sauce pan and add 1 tablespoon of the herb mixture for every cup of water. Bring to a rolling boil. Allow the herbs to simmer for 10 minutes. Turn off the heat and let sit for another 5 minutes. Strain out the herbs. Be sure to take at least three deep inhalations of the tea before you begin drinking it: the first breath through the mouth, the second through the nose, and the third through the mouth again. Add honey if desired, and sip.

DOSE / TIMING / DURATION

Drink 4–6 cups per day as needed until symptoms subside for up to 2 weeks. If cough and other symptoms worsen, do not respond to home therapies, are accompanied by a high fever or continue for more than 3 weeks, it is important to consult with a healthcare provider.

Osha root and cherry bark are to be used during acute illness, for a limited period of time, not as ongoing therapy.

BENEFITS

This tastes like medicine, but it is well worth it! Strongly antiviral and immune stimulating, this tea helps dry out and expectorate excessive mucus in the lungs. It is also warming and promotes sweating, an important route of elimination. It is high in aromatic oils, making it useful to the lungs when inhaled.

INDICATIONS

Useful for both upper and lower respiratory tract infections; sinus congestion, bronchitis, and pneumonia, especially when excessive mucus is present.

CAUTIONS

- Wild cherry bark should not be used during pregnancy due to its teratogenic effects.

- Wild cherry bark should generally not be taken for extended periods of time.

- Oregon grape root should not be used during pregnancy because it contains several compounds that stimulate the uterus.

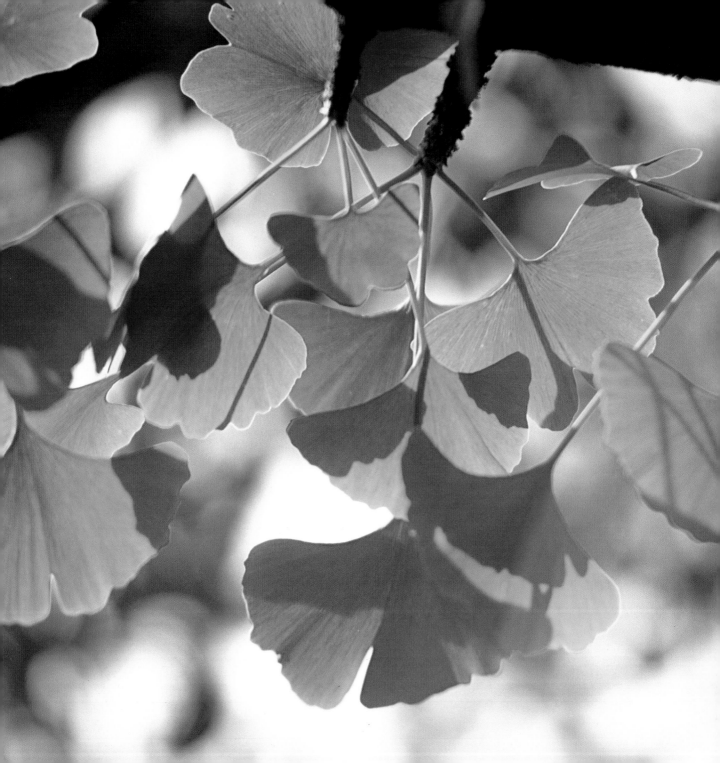

Chapter 9

Strong Healthy Heart

Cardiovascular health depends on a strong pump—the heart—and clear blood vessels. Most diseases of the cardiovascular system begin as the vessels become blocked and hardened. This leads to high blood pressure, weakening of the heart muscles, and eventually congestive heart failure. Atherosclerosis, the buildup of fatty plaques on the inside of artery walls leads to a narrowing of the blood vessels and a hardening of their otherwise elastic walls. This elasticity is important in that it allows for them to expand to take the large quantity of blood that is pumped out of the heart. The body, in its elegant design, has the more elastic vessels closest to the heart to allow for this, while the smaller, less elastic vessels are more distant from the heart.

As the vessels become blocked or narrowed as plaque builds up inside them, they lose their elasticity and the pressure within them increases and an increase in blood pressure occurs—hypertension. Next, pieces of plaque break off and begin moving through the vascular system. The emboli (as the piece of released plaque is called) moves through the brain, a stroke occurs. Because balance in the nervous system affects the rhythm of the contracting heart and the responsiveness of the vessels, the first line of defense in cardiovascular health, as with all systems of our bodies, is to respond to stress appropriately. See Chapter 2 for details on dealing with stress.

Herbs that promote circulation and dilate vessels: hawthorn, ginger, ginkgo, cayenne, garlic, and lemon balm.

Blood thinning herbs that decrease platelet aggregation and clot formation: garlic, ginkgo, ginger, and cayenne.

Herbs that balance the nervous system and its effect on the blood vessels: motherwort and lemon balm.

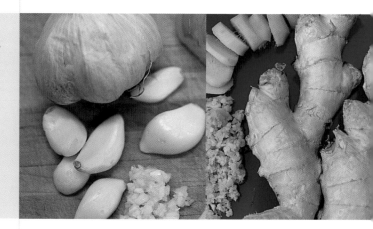

smaller and smaller vessels until it finally gets to a vessel that is too small for it to move through, and it becomes lodged, blocking the vessel. The severity of this situation varies depending on the location of the blockage. If it occurs in a leg, you may experience cramping pain, numbness, or some loss of function. If this occurs in a coronary artery of the heart, it can cause loss of function of some of the heart muscle leading to a heart attack. If it occurs in an artery to

Herbs support healthy cardiovascular function in many ways. Herbs can be nutritive to the cardiac tissue and vasculature, they can balance the nervous system and its effects on the heart and vessels, they can thin the blood, and they can promote circulation. The herbs discussed in this book are generally safe and there is little danger of misuse or adverse reactions. However, every individual is unique and may have responses to an herb that are not common.

> Nutritive cardiovascular herbs that strengthen the heart muscles and blood vessels: hawthorn, ginkgo, and motherwort.

If you have a cardiovascular condition or are taking medications, it is best to work with a healthcare practitioner knowledgeable about herbs rather than to self-prescribe.

One of the best ways to promote a healthy heart is to include cardiovascular herbs regularly in your diet. Use cayenne pepper, garlic, and ginger frequently in your cooking. It may seem simple and folksy to make such a suggestion, but these herbs have been scientifically shown to dilate blood vessels, decrease platelet aggregation, and decrease the formation of fatty plaques and thrombi. If nature intended for us to take in enormous amounts of these herbs, as is possible with those available in capsules, it would have made them milder to the tongue. The very fact that these plants have bite is an indication that we should use them in moderate quantities.

Hawthorn

Hawthorn is a wonderful nutritive tonic that would be beneficial to include in your diet daily. Historically hawthorn has been used in jams and jellies as a regular part of the diet. The Sweet Heart-Ease Tea™ is a wonderful and simple way to include hawthorn in your diet.

I remember fondly my first introduction to hawthorn. I was a student at the National College of Naturopathic Medicine, taking an elective course called Northwest Herbs. This course was held in the fall, winter, and spring, and was our opportunity to have hands-on learning with the herbs. In this class, we drank herbal teas, made herbal extracts for internal consumption and topical application, and learned how to harvest herbs, how to process them fresh, how to dry them, and how to identify them in the wild. That was the best part—our field trips to identify and wild-harvest herbs.

One foggy, damp fall morning (we call it "dry rain" in Portland—not really raining enough to warrant an umbrella) a group of 10–12 of us ventured out to Oaks Bottom, a marshy park by the river. Our guide was Judy Bluehorse Skelton, a Native American. Judy is very simple in her manner, not at all flashy. I think it is that quality that allows a beautiful

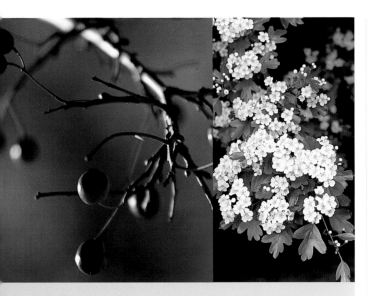

HAWTHORN BERRY GLYCERITE

Hawthorn berries can be made into a glycerite quite simply. Around November 1, hawthorn berries are usually ripe and abundant. Take a small jar with you as you go out to wild-harvest hawthorn berries from an abundant, unpolluted area or perhaps from the tree in your backyard. Fill 1/3 of the jar with carefully chosen, healthy hawthorn berries. When you get home, fill another 1/3 of the jar with pure vegetable glycerine. Cover, and shake daily for 2 weeks. After this period of time, strain and place the glycerite in a dark-colored bottle. You can then take a teaspoon of your hawthorn glycerite daily.

strength and clarity to shine through her. On this particular walk, we tasted the hips of wild rose bushes and we came across a St. John's wort plant growing out of the rocks by the side of the path that still had some seeds in its pods for us to gather, take home, and freeze until spring when we could plant them in the ground.

But the purpose of our field trip that day was to make a hawthorn glycerite—hawthorn berries extracted and preserved in vegetable glycerine. So we stepped off the path into a muddy, almost marshy orchard-like spot. Judy led us to a small grove of hawthorn trees. Hawthorn trees without their flowers and leaves have a sort of scraggly look; they look almost broken with their thorny branches going off in unexpected directions.

We stood around the hawthorn trees as Judy told us about them and began to harvest the berries one at a time, placing them directly into our glass jars with their inch of glycerin waiting for the fruit. As Judy spoke about the qualities of hawthorn, a kind of magical presence filled the air. The moment felt very full. As she spoke, thoughts of my father came to my mind. The more she spoke, the more strongly I felt connected to him. As I reached my hand up to the tree to pick each berry, I felt that I was being guided to just the right ones, as if there was an energetic pull

Sweet Heart-Ease™ Tea

INGREDIENTS

1 part Hawthorn berry
1 part Hawthorn flower and leaf
1/6 part Stevia leaf (or to taste)

INSTRUCTIONS

Using your favorite tea-making tool (tea pot, French press, infusing basket, or tea ball), add 1 heaping teaspoon of the herb mixture to each cup of just boiled water. Cover and let sit for approximately 5 minutes. Pour the tea into a cup, straining out the herbs (or remove the infusing basket or tea ball), and drink.

DOSE / TIMING / DURATION

Drink 3–4 cups daily. Hawthorn is best when taken on a long-term basis. It is a tonifying, nutritive herb that has historically been used as an herbal food.

BENEFITS

Hawthorn is the premier cardiac tonic. It strengthens the contraction of the heart muscle, normalizes blood pressure, increases vascular integrity, and prevents free-radical damage. Hawthorn is anti-inflammatory due to inhibition of histamine, prostaglandins, and leukotrienes. Stevia leaf is believed to aid in blood-sugar regulation and to have an anti-hypertensive action; it adds a sweet taste and is safe for most diabetics.

INDICATIONS

Beneficial for most conditions of the heart and vascular system: arteriosclerosis, hypertension, hypotension, venous stasis, congestive heart failure, cardiac arrhythmias, valvular murmur and regurgitation, angina, asthma, diabetes, high cholesterol, inflammation, intermittent claudication, and Raynaud's disease.

CAUTIONS

- There is very little toxic potential with long-term use of hawthorn.

- Hawthorn potentiates the actions of cardiac glycoside medications such as digitoxin and digoxin. If you are taking cardiac medications, their levels should be monitored regularly because the use of hawthorn may allow for a decrease in their doses.

Remember: It's a good idea to take a break from any herb that you use daily on an ongoing basis. Consider taking a 2-week break every 3–4 months.

to one berry instead of another. The feeling was so strong that I finally looked at Judy and said, "I feel like I'm picking each one of these for my father!" There was a silence as Judy's eyes got even brighter. Then she said, in her very simple way, "Yes, there's a lot of father's energy here right now." She smiled as the silence filled the space around us. Then following her directions, we put the lids on our jars, some of us gave them their first good shake, and we continued on our walk.

That first sweet hawthorn glycerite was ready by January, and I gave it to my father for his birthday. He is not a person who is very familiar with herbs or natural medicine, but he somehow knew the special-ness of the herbal extract of hawthorn that I gave him. He took it religiously every day. He even carried it with him when he traveled. No matter which city I met him in, I would see it sitting on the bathroom counter or he would pull it out of his travel bag to show me how much he had left.

Hawthorn is said to nourish the heart. Physiologi-cally it is known to literally nourish the heart muscle to increase its strength of contraction. But many herbalists also talk about the way that hawthorn nour-ishes our heart center—the energetic heart—the one that opens when we feel love and breaks when love is lost. And here it was, strengthening the connection between the heart of father and daughter.

By the time my father finished the hawthorn glycerite, I had started my company The Art of Health, Inc. One of my first products, Sweet Heart-Ease Tea™ on page 113, is made of hawthorn flower, leaf, and berries and sweetened with the herb stevia (inspired by Lakota herbalist Debra Francis, N.D.— Beautiful Little Dancing Crow). Now my father drinks this tea every day and it continues to nourish both of our hearts.

Other Herbs

The other herbs discussed in this chapter can be taken in the form of a tincture, tea, or even a vinegar. Motherwort and lemon balm make an excellent vinegar that relieves anxiety that is accompanied by heart palpitations. This can be taken in water before meals, to support digestion, as well. See the direc-tions in Chapter 13 on making herbal vinegars.

The Simple Clarity Tea recipe that follows fea-tures the cardiovascular benefits of ginkgo, lemon balm, and goto kola, the last also furnishing nour-ishment to the adrenal glands, the body's primary stress-response organ.

There are other herbs that are very useful in the treatment of heart disease that I do not discuss in this

Simple Clarity™—A Circulatory Tea

INGREDIENTS

1 part Ginkgo leaf
1 part Gotu kola herb
1 part Lemon balm leaf
1/2 part Lavender buds
1/6 part Stevia leaf

INSTRUCTIONS

Using your favorite tea-making tool (tea pot, French press, infusing basket, or tea ball), add 1 heaping teaspoon of the herb mixture to each cup of just boiled water. Cover and let sit for approximately 5 minutes. Pour the tea into a cup, straining out the herbs (or remove the infusing basket or tea ball), inhale the tea's aroma, and sip slowly.

DOSE / TIMING / DURATION

Drink up to 4 cups daily.

BENEFITS

Stimulates circulation and increases blood flow to the brain and throughout the body by dilating the blood vessels. Decreases platelet aggregation and thrombosis, preventing strokes. Has antioxidant properties, decreasing cellular damage caused by free radicals. Supports the body's ability to respond appropriately to stress by nourishing the adrenal glands.

INDICATIONS

High blood pressure, cerebral arteriosclerosis, atherosclerosis, intermittent claudication, Raynaud's disease, and varicose veins.

CAUTIONS

- Gotu kola, lavender, and lemon balm can bring on menses, so should not be used during pregnancy unless supervised by a qualified healthcare provider.

- Ginkgo should not be used prior to surgery or by people with hemophilia.

book because they are potentially toxic. These include lily of the valley, which increases circulation to the coronary arteries; fox glove (*Digitalis*), which supports slow but forceful contractions of the heart muscle; and hellebore (veratrum), which lowers the blood pressure and heart rate. If you are interested in exploring the uses of these stronger-acting herbs, consult a Naturopathic physician for guidance.

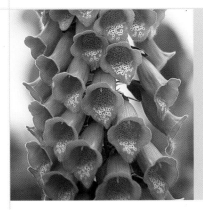

Fox glove

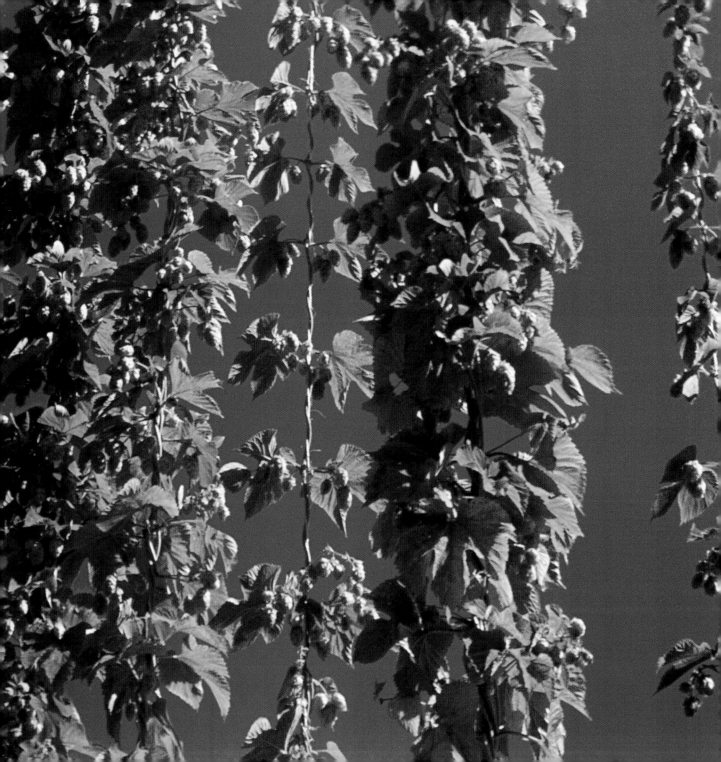

Chapter 10

Freedom to Choose: Breaking Unhealthy Habits

Many habits that are potentially harmful tend to have an addictive effect, for example, smoking cigarettes, drinking caffeinated beverages, and eating chocolate or excessive amounts of sugar. The moderate intake of these potentially unhealthy substances may be fine but becomes problematic when the addictive substance consumes us. When a significant part of our resources (time, money, and energy) goes into acquiring, consuming, or thinking about any of these substances, their level of consumption is not promoting balance or our highest state of well-being. When the substance or the desire for the substance takes over, we have lost our freedom to choose and are being controlled by it. It is then necessary to change our relationship to the substance. Often this means eliminating it completely, at least for a while. This is not always easy because we, as a whole person, have become used to it in many ways.

Many books on health provide a list of dos and don'ts. They tell us what healthy behavior is and is not, which foods are healthy and which are not, which substances are good for us and which are not, and which lifestyle habits are healthy and which are not. From these, we could easily get the impression that, if only we were perfect, more disciplined, and more motivated, we could then follow this list of dos and don'ts and be healthy. The problem is that living by these lists can cause a feeling of restriction. We then go through life seeing all that we *can't* do or have or eat. A feeling of deprivation sets in. Some people are able to create very strict rules for themselves and live by them. But others will fall off the wagon again and again and again and feel like failures. Is setting up a situation so that you cannot succeed healthy? Is labeling yourself a failure healthy? I don't think so. It does not promote wellness from within. It does not create a state of balance. It is not a framework that promotes the expansion of our awareness and ability to operate with increased flow within our environment.

From another perspective, there are foods, habits, and lifestyles that generally promote health and those that generally tend to place stress on the body. Too much of the latter overwhelms the body's self-healing mechanisms and leads to imbalance or, in the extreme case, a disease of some kind. We need to find a healthy balance. Sometimes that means using a restrictive approach by eliminating a food or substance that is problematic. Depending on the potential for negative effects of the food or substance, we may need to avoid it indefinitely or we may need only a temporary break from it to bring the body back to a state in which the homeostatic mechanisms are restored, one in which the substance can be introduced and enjoyed occasionally without negatively affecting health and wellness.

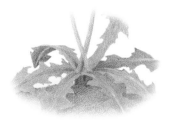

Breaking the Addictive Cycle

Herbs can be used to help us break these addictive cycles and restore our freedom to choose. The feelings of withdrawal that we experience when we eliminate a substance to which we are accustomed to can include nervous irritability, shakiness, agitation and anxiety, and increased sensitivity to light and noise. There are wonderful herbs that address those very symptoms: chamomile, oats, skullcap, peppermint, catnip, and hops. This particular combination of herbs is, in fact, based on a formula originally created at an addictions center to support the cessation of smoking. I like to use these herbs as a tea (New Leaf Tea™) because drinking the cup of tea in and of itself acts as a replacement for activity we are trying to eliminate (smoking a cigarette, drinking a cup of coffee, eating a piece of chocolate, etc.). So, in addition to the herbs in the tea calming the nerves, relieving the craving, and releasing muscle tension, drinking the tea gives us a pleasant substitution for the undesirable activity. See also the Castor Oil Pack Treatment later in this chapter.

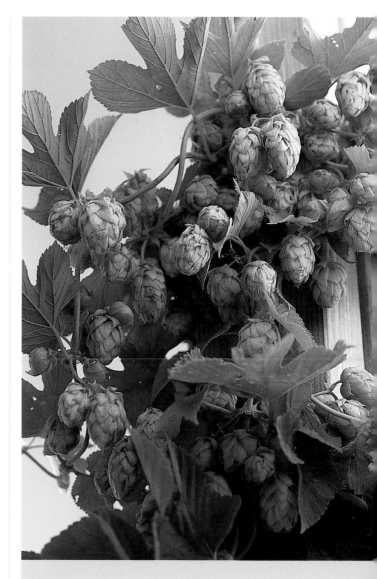

Hops

New Leaf Tea™

INGREDIENTS

> 1 part German Chamomile flowers
> 2 parts Oatstraw and/or milky oat seeds
> 1/2 part Skullcap
> 1/2 part Peppermint
> 1/2 part Catnip
> 1/6 part Hops

INSTRUCTIONS

Using your favorite tea-making tool (tea pot, French press, infusing basket, or tea ball), add 1 heaping teaspoon of the herb mixture to each cup of just boiled water. Cover and let sit for approximately 5 minutes. Pour the tea into a cup, straining out the herbs (or remove the infusing basket or tea ball), inhale the tea's aroma, and sip slowly.

DOSE / TIMING / DURATION

Drink up to 4–6 cups daily as needed. The tea can be used as a substitute for a cigarette or coffee break or taken throughout the day to prevent the craving for these substances from coming on.

BENEFITS

The herbs in this formula have been used to help hundreds of people stop smoking. They are anti-addictive. They calm and soothe the nervousness, agitation, and irritability that accompany the elimination of addictive substances such as nicotine, alcohol, and caffeine.

INDICATIONS

A supportive tool when you are ready to make a change such as the cessation of smoking or elimination of caffeinated substances or alcoholic beverages.

CAUTIONS

- Chamomile may cause an allergic reaction in susceptible individuals, which may involve a skin rash, difficulty breathing, hives, or other hypersensitivity reactions. You should avoid chamomile if you know that you are allergic to plants in the Asteraceae/Compositae family. If you are unsure, introduce chamomile into your herbal repertoire carefully. If no adverse reaction occurs, you should feel free to use it as desired.

- Peppermint and catnip can bring on menses and should only be used during pregnancy under the guidance of a healthcare practitioner familiar with the use of herbs.

A Sugar Substitute

Another way that herbs can support us in making a change is to act as substitutes for the unhealthy substance. For example, if we are trying to give up sugar, the herb stevia can be of enormous use. Stevia, also known as the sweet plant of Paraguay, is, in its natural form, 30 times sweeter than sugar but has no calories and does not raise the blood sugar. Stevia has been used in native cultures for over 100 years. In 1954, researchers in Japan began to study it seriously. It is used in Japan extensively to sweeten pickles, dried foods, soy sauce, fruit juices, soft drinks, frozen deserts, gum, and diet foods.

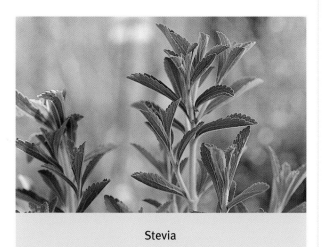

Stevia

Stevia is not only a sweet plant that is less harmful than sugar and artificial sweeteners, but there is research that shows stevia has a positive impact on the body. It has been studied for its potential beneficial effects for diabetics in regulating blood sugar. Stevia has been shown to retard the growth of plaque in the mouth and to be anti-carcinogenic. Stevia leaf can be included whole in a tea that you blend yourself, or you can by it powdered or in liquid drops. These forms make it easy to use stevia to sweeten homemade baked goods or your favorite beverages, such as teas or lemonade.

Cleansing the System

Another important factor in changing addictive patterns is to eliminate the buildup of the offending substance from the body. This will naturally happen over time, but as long as the substance remains in the body there will be a tendency to continue to crave it and it will be more difficult to stay away from it. It is therefore extremely useful to promote detoxification through as many pathways as possible. Herbs are helpful in promoting detoxification by cleansing the liver and kidneys and by promoting elimination through the digestive tract. In Chapter 7, you will find my favorite recipe for supporting liver detoxification,

Liver Cleansing Tea. The herbs in this tea can be used as everyday support or as part of a cleansing regimen.

Another way to cleanse the liver and help eliminate toxins from the body is by using a castor oil pack. This is a relaxing, self-nurturing treatment with countless benefits. Most often applied as a pack placed over the abdomen, the oil is absorbed into circulation, providing a cleansing, nutritive, and relaxing treatment. Having personally tried to give up caffeine and sugar both with and without the use of castor oil packs, I highly recommend them any time you eliminate a food or substance from your diet and therefore your body. For me, it completely eliminated the symptoms of withdrawal, such as headache and irritability. Now I wouldn't even think about trying to make such a change without the use of castor oil packs.

One Step at a Time

Any time you choose to drink an herbal tea instead of coffee or another addictive substance, you are taking a positive step toward the expression of your freedom to choose and create total well-being. No step should be belittled; each one is huge. Be careful not to ascribe failure if you don't make that choice today. This is a gradual process, one of experimentation and of learning what is best for you. If you indulge, it doesn't mean you have failed. Every choice you make is part of a path to transforming yourself. You may never completely eliminate sugar, and there may be no reason to do so. But consciously choosing to eat sugar on occasion is different than being controlled by it, with every hour of the day spent thinking about where you are going to get more. Or perhaps you don't think about it all the time, but you get every cold that comes along and you have trouble shaking it off because your immune system is depleted due to chronic or excessive sugar consumption. Breaking addictive patterns is not a matter of perfectly following the rules, so that if you don't you have failed. It's not all or nothing. Each step is one more on the pathway to optimal health. The simple act of picking up this book and reading it is one of those choices you have made to thrive instead of just survive.

Castor Oil Pack Treatment

MATERIALS

Castor oil
Plastic sheet (or plastic wrap or
   a plastic trash bag)
1 yard white cotton or wool flannel
Heating pad or hot water bottle
Old sheet
Wool blanket
Solution of 3 tablespoons of baking
   soda to 1 quart water (optional)

INSTRUCTIONS

Fold the flannel into three thicknesses to fit over your entire abdomen. Soak the flannel with enough castor oil to fully saturate the cloth.

Decide where you will lie down. On this surface, spread out a wool blanket, and cover it with an old sheet, an old towel, and a large sheet of plastic. These will hold in the heat and prevent staining.

Lie on your back on your covered blanket and place the oil-soaked flannel over your abdomen. Wrap yourself in the plastic sheet and towel, and place a heating pad or hot water bottle on top of the towel. Then wrap the sheet and wool blanket around you.

Leave pack on for 60–90 minutes. During this time, rest quietly. You may want to listen to quiet music or meditate.

When time is up, unwrap yourself. If the oil bothers you, wash with a solution of 3 tablespoons of baking soda to 1 quart water.

Store the pack in a large zip-lock bag. The oil and pack can be reused several times, adding more oil as needed to keep the pack well saturated. Replace the pack after it begins to change color. This may occur in days, weeks, or months.

TIMING / DURATION

The castor oil pack will be most effective when left on for 60–90 minutes and done for 4 or 5 consecutive days per week for 1 month.

BENEFITS

The castor bean (*Oleum ricini*) also known as Palma Christi, has been shown to facilitate elimination through the digestive and urinary tracts, improve intestinal absorption of nutrients, dissolve lesions, reduce inflammation, relieve pain, improve coordination of the nervous system, and improve function in many vital organs.

INDICATIONS

Castor oil packs are recommended in numerous circumstances such as cleansing and detoxification regimens, inflamed joints, constipation and other intestinal disorders, PMS and other conditions caused by hormonal imbalance, liver disorders, headache, gallbladder conditions, and nonmalignant growths such as uterine fibroids and ovarian cysts.

CAUTIONS

Castor oil packs should not be used during pregnancy, with an open wound, or during menstruation.

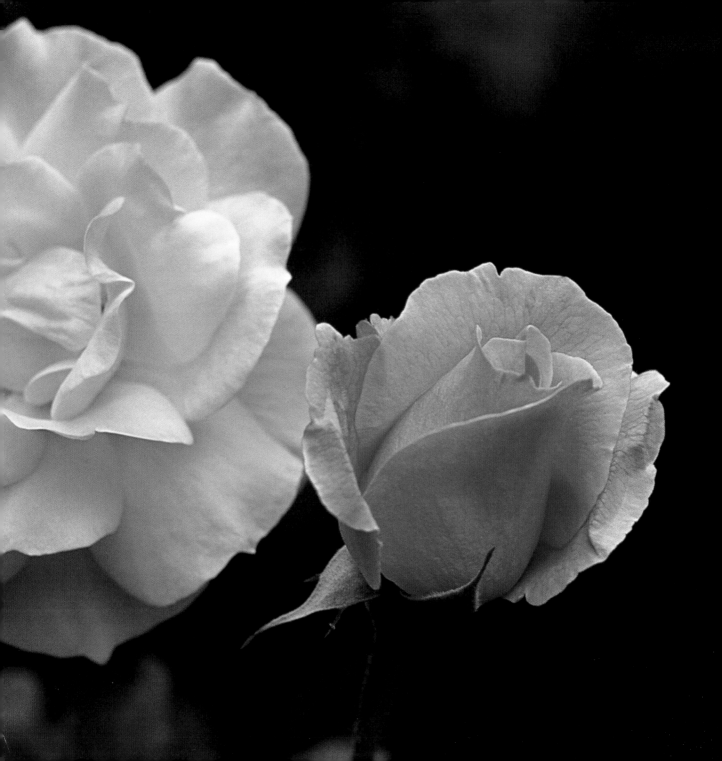

Chapter 11

Healthy Happy Children

The great strength of natural therapies lies in their ability to keep us healthy, to prevent illness. Unfortunately many adults are introduced to natural therapies, including the use of herbs, only after they have become seriously ill and have exhausted all the allopathic therapies. As a last resort, they may seek out a Naturopathic physician or another holistic practitioner. With children, however, natural therapeutic approaches have the opportunity to shine because their conditions are generally acute and their self-healing know-how (unlike the adults') is uncorrupted by years of compensation and adaptation to life's stressors.

Nutrition

Of course the most basic therapy for children and adults is good nutrition. Breast-feeding plays a vital role in the development of the child's immune system. Proper introduction of foods makes sure that the child's immunity is not overly taxed while it is still developing. Herbs can be included as food to make sure the diet contains a wealth of the plant nutrients available and necessary for the functioning of the human body. For example, nettles or dandelion greens can be steamed, pureed, and mixed with more common foods such as carrots, sweet potatoes, and spinach.

Herbal Therapies to Restore Balance

Herbs can also help maintain the health of children by supporting them through acute illnesses such as a colic, ear infections, colds, and coughs. Herbal therapies are extremely useful in these instances because they support the body's natural effort to restore balance, instead of suppressing it as do many of the over-the-counter medications. The use of such suppressive medications over time can lead to a weakened immune system, leading to further illness.

COLIC AND TEETHING

Colic involves episodes of crying and fussiness that do not respond to comforting. The infant may pull his or her legs up, the abdomen may be hard, and they may be relieved by passing gas. Colic generally occurs in infants between 2 weeks and 12 weeks of age. The cause is unclear. It is possible that it is a result of disorganization of peristalsis or autonomic nervous system function (this is the portion of

TEETHING PAIN

For teething pain, massage the baby gently with lavender oil. Massage the hand, including a point at the back of the hand at the end of the crease between the thumb and forefinger. This is a Chinese acupressure point used for centuries as dental anesthesia. See also the Teething and Colic Tea in this chapter.

the nervous system that includes the parasympathetic nervous system; see Chapter 4). Colic may also be a result of tension, overfeeding, or an intestinal allergy—often to cow's milk.

Treatments

Some useful home remedies for colic include massaging dilute peppermint oil onto the child's abdomen. The peppermint essential oil can be added to any fixed oil such as almond oil or castor oil, which has its own pain-relieving qualities. Chamomile or other herbs such as fennel, ginger, peppermint, catnip can be taken internally as a tea to relieve the discomfort. See one example of Teething and Colic Tea on page 130. If the child is nursing, the mother should avoid caffeine, chocolate, cow's milk, and any foods to which she knows she is allergic or sensitive. The mother can also drink fennel and fenugreek tea, which will make its way to the baby via her breast milk. Constitutional Home Hydrotherapy Treatment (on page 128) applied over the baby's abdomen will be very soothing. You can even soak the towels (actually washcloths work best for infants) in chamomile tea or sprinkle them with a little lavender or peppermint essential oil before applying them to the baby's belly.

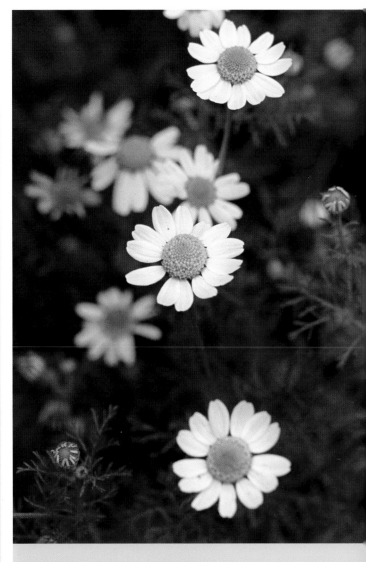

Chamomile

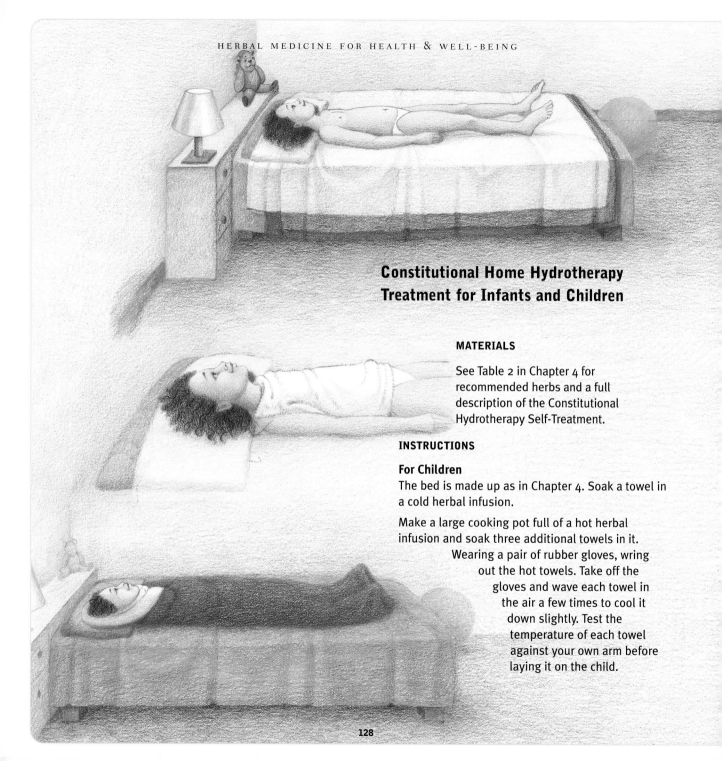

Constitutional Home Hydrotherapy Treatment for Infants and Children

MATERIALS

See Table 2 in Chapter 4 for recommended herbs and a full description of the Constitutional Hydrotherapy Self-Treatment.

INSTRUCTIONS

For Children

The bed is made up as in Chapter 4. Soak a towel in a cold herbal infusion.

Make a large cooking pot full of a hot herbal infusion and soak three additional towels in it. Wearing a pair of rubber gloves, wring out the hot towels. Take off the gloves and wave each towel in the air a few times to cool it down slightly. Test the temperature of each towel against your own arm before laying it on the child.

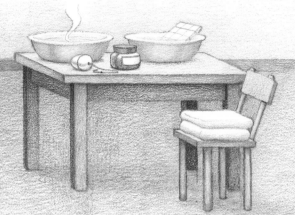

Lay two of the hot towels (one on top of the other) across his or her chest and abdomen. Close the sheet and blankets around the child snugly and wait 5 minutes. Unwrap the child and remove the towels.

Place a fresh hot towel on the child for 30 seconds to 1 minute.

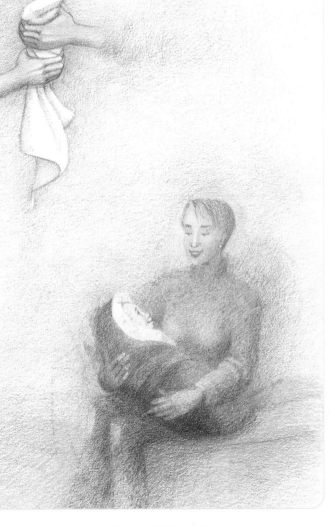

Replace this hot towel with the cold towel that has been wrung out well. Again, wrap the child tightly. And let him or her rest for at least 10 minutes or until the cold towel feels warmed. Unwrap the child and have him or her roll over onto the abdomen. Repeat the steps, this time laying the towels on the child's back.

For Infants
To give the home hydrotherapy treatment to an infant, warm the baby in a bath. Then apply a cold washcloth to his or her chest and abdomen, wrap him or her in wool blankets, and rock gently.

BENEFITS, INDICATIONS, AND CAUTIONS

See Table 2 in Chapter 4.

Teething and Colic Tea

INGREDIENTS

Chamomile
Skullcap
Lemon balm
Lavender

Use equal parts of each herb.

INSTRUCTIONS

Using your favorite tea-making tool (tea pot, French press, infusing basket, or tea ball), add 1 heaping teaspoon of the herb mixture to each cup of just boiled water. Cover and let sit for approximately 5 minutes. Pour the tea into a cup, straining out the herbs (or remove the infusing basket or tea ball). If needed, add one of the sweeteners recommended for children.

As a Tea

To give herbal teas to an infant use a dropper, making sure the tea has cooled to room temperature.

As an External Treatment

To use as an external treatment for teething pain, soak a soft cotton cloth in the tea and give it to the infant to chew on. Simply by holding the cloth, the infant will benefit from the soothing aroma and possibly absorb some of the herbs through the skin (depending on how much contact is made).

DOSE / TIMING / DURATION

Drink 1–4 cups per day.

BENEFITS

Antispasmodic, relieves gas and bloating, pain relieving, and mildly sedating,

INDICATIONS

Pain, discomfort, and irritability from teething or colic.

CAUTIONS

Make sure the tea has cooled before giving to an infant either internally or externally.

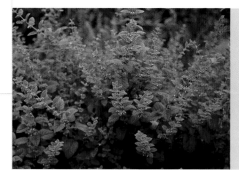

Lemon balm

CONSTIPATION IN CHILDREN

In cases of constipation in children, nutritional causes should first be considered. In babies, it is often the result of dietary changes such as changing from breast milk to formula or early introduction of solid foods. In older children, constipation is likely to be caused by a food allergy or sensitivity. Identification of food allergens and avoidance of them will generally clear up the problem as well as generally strengthening the child's immune system and promoting greater health. Increased water intake and foods high in fiber such as oatmeal and apples are also helpful. Herbal teas can support regular bowel movements. For kids, try fennel, catnip, or the Liver Cleansing Tea (containing alterative herbs) in Chapter 7.

The treatment of food allergies or sensitivities is beyond the scope of this book. Naturopathic physicians are an excellent resource for treatment of food allergies. To find a Naturopathic physician, contact an accredited Naturopathic college for assistance in finding a physician near you (see the Epilogue at the end of the book).

EAR INFECTIONS

Otitis media is the most common problem in young children. It is the result of a bacterial infection of the middle ear. The use of pacifiers can lead to increased occurrence of ear infections. This is because the constant sucking causes a negative pressure in the ears that keeps them from draining properly. The buildup of fluid creates an environment hospitable for bacterial growth. Allergies can also lead to ear infections because they can cause the eustachian tubes to swell, again preventing proper drainage; also, constant sniffling can again create negative pressure and decreased drainage.

Acute otitis may be treated with ear drops made from mullein and garlic. Care must be taken not to use these drops in the ear of a child whose eardrum (tympanic membrane) is perforated. A physician can see this in his or her examination. If there is perforation, or if a perforation seems likely to occur in the near future, a poultice can be used safely. Comfrey, garlic, and ginger are all good choices and should be applied with dry heat (see Chapter 12). Echinacea or larix can be used internally to stimulate the immune response. Children's formulations of these herbs are readily available at health food stores. Or try making your own echinacea glycerite using echinacea root

Cough and Cold Syrup for Children

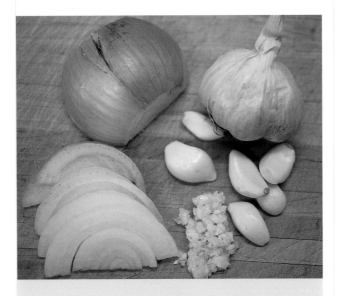

Onion and garlic

INGREDIENTS

An onion or a bulb of garlic
Honey

INSTRUCTIONS

Slice the onion or crush the whole bulb of garlic and cover with honey. Bake until soft. Strain the syrup.

DOSE / TIMING / DURATION

Take a teaspoonful of the syrup up to 4 times per day during an infection. If symptoms worsen, do not respond to home therapies, are accompanied by a high fever, or continue for more than 3 weeks, consult with a healthcare provider.

BENEFITS

The syrup is a pleasant-tasting way to ingest the anti-microbial and immune-stimulating properties of garlic and onions. The honey also has anti-microbial properties and acts as an expectorant. Baking draws out the mucilage in the onions and garlic, which supports thinning thick mucus and soothing inflamed respiratory passageways.

INDICATIONS

Coughs associated with cold, flu, or bronchitis.

CAUTIONS

Garlic consumption should be monitored in individuals taking blood-thinning medications or undergoing surgery.

from your garden (see Chapter 13). As always, the therapies in this book are not meant as a substitution for a diagnosis from a licensed physician but to provide information for you to apply when you already know what's wrong.

Also effective for treating ear aches is the Warming Sock Treatment (see Chapter 3), which is pain relieving and immune supporting. In addition, an alternating hot and cold compress treatment over the ear with circulatory and calming essential oils, such as peppermint, in water can be used (see Chapter 12).

Herbs work very effectively in children to address allergic or viral catarrh (nasal stuffiness). For allergic stuffiness, try nettles, ginger, peppermint, fennel, and eyebright in teas. The same herbs can be used for viral infections with the addition of garlic. To make garlic palatable for children, try the preceding recipe for a garlic/honey cough and cold syrup.

UPPER RESPIRATORY INFECTIONS

For upper respiratory infections, many of the same treatments discussed for ear infections are appropriate. Reduce sugar intake to ease the burden on the immune system, and use herbs such as echinacea, mullein, red clover, osha, garlic, and licorice to support the immune system. Drinking warm fluids

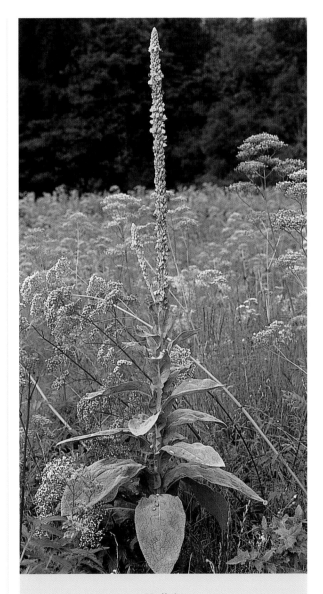

Mullein

Table 5

Herbs for Calming Baths

HERBS	BENEFITS	INDICATIONS	CAUTIONS
Chamomile flowers	Relieves muscle spasm, relieves pain, mildly sedating	Restlessness with irritability or anxiety	Individuals allergic to plants in the Compositae/Asteracea family may react to chamomile
Lavender buds	Calming, relieves muscle spasm, mildly sedating	Headaches, muscle spasms, agitation, nervous exhaustion, insomnia	No contraindications for external use
Rose petals	Soothes inflamed skin, calming yet uplifting, relieves muscle spasm, revitalizing	Insomnia, grief, depression, muscle spasm, stress, tension headache, fatigue	No contraindications for external use
Lemon balm leaf	Calming and soothing to the nerves, mildly sedating, relaxes muscles	Anxiety or irritability with restlessness, palpitations, and headache	No contraindications for external use

will help open up congested passageways; the Warming Sock Treatment (Chapter 3) will keep them open through the night. All the treatments discussed in Chapter 5 are applicable here, with the doses adjusted to the size of the child. Adult dosages are based on an average-size adult, approximately 150 pounds. For a child, or someone who weighs significantly more or less than 150 pounds, the following rule can be used to calculate dose:

$$\text{Child's weight in pounds} \div 150 \text{ pounds}$$
$$= \text{Fraction of the adult dose}$$

Herbal baths are also very effective for calming sick children at bedtime, as is the Warming Sock Treatment (Chapter 3). These treatments are very soothing to children and adults alike.

WARTS

Warts are common, mildly contagious skin lesions caused by a virus. They are more common in older children. They may itch or bleed, especially if the child picks at them. Effective treatment for warts varies quite a bit from one person to another. Because they are caused by a virus, an anti-viral therapy such

Calming Herbal Baths

MATERIALS

Chamomile flowers
Lavender buds
Rose petals
Lemon balm leaf
Stocking or sock

Use 1 cup of any of the dried herbs listed (or a mixture of any two or more of them).

INSTRUCTIONS

Place herbs in a stocking or thin sock and knot it at the end to make an herbal bath bag. Begin filling the bathtub, or sink for infants, with hot water, letting the water from the faucet fall over the herbal bath bag. When the bath is approximately 1/3 full with the herbally infused water, continue to fill with cooler water. Monitor the temperature of the water to make it comfortable for bathing. Another technique is to fill the tub completely with hot water then let it cool to a comfortable temperature. The longer you have hot water running over the herbal bath bag, the stronger the herbal infusion will be. Squeeze the herbal bath bag periodically to increase the strength of the infusion.

DOSE / TIMING / DURATION

This bath can be used as the daily bathing ritual or when a child is fussy, experiencing pain or discomfort, or is overly energized.

BENEFITS, INDICATIONS, AND CAUTIONS

See Table 5 on page 134.

Warts Away!

MATERIALS

1/2-ounce bottle cold-pressed Castor oil
7 drops Peppermint essential oil
Band-Aid

INSTRUCTIONS

Add 7 drops peppermint essential oil to a 1/2-oz bottle of castor oil. Turn bottle 180 degrees to the left and then to the right several times to ensure the two ingredients are well mixed. Cover the padded portion of a Band-Aid with the oil mixture and place over the wart.

DOSE / TIMING / DURATION

The oil-soaked bandage can be left on day and night, but should be changed each day. The wart may resolve within a few days or it may take several weeks. If treatment time is prolonged, be sure to give the area breaks from being bandaged. (I have seen it take 3–4 months for plantar warts that did not respond to other treatments to heal in adults—so be patient.)

BENEFITS

Dissolves and removes lesions, pain relieving, increases circulation to the skin, and boosts the immune response.

INDICATIONS

Warts anywhere on the body.

CAUTIONS

- If skin irritation occurs, decrease the amount of peppermint essential oil used.

- Peppermint essential oil should not be applied to the skin undiluted.

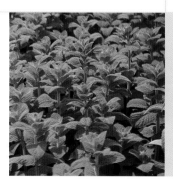

Mint

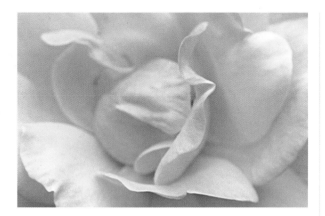

stevia leaf to your herb mixture. Another approach is to mix the herbal tea or extract with fruit juice, or to add dried orange peels or cinnamon to your herbal teas to make them sweeter and more palatable for children.

Another way to make herbs more palatable for kids is to add a little pleasant-tasting essential oil to a liquid herbal extract, for example, bitter orange, peppermint, or fennel. This is a very good option if it meets the child's taste standards because sugars, even honey, can suppress the immune system and promote the growth of bacteria and viruses.

You can also purchase a fun straw with loops and fun characters on it that is to be used only for herbal teas. Or try freezing an herbal tea in ice cube trays with a tooth pick in the center of each cube. The child can then have several "popsicles" a day. This is especially nice in the case of a sore throat.

as garlic is sometimes useful. Garlic can be taken internally or applied as a compress directly to the wart. Castor oil can be applied to a Band-Aid and placed over the wart, as in the preceding recipe. Another treatment for warts is to apply the white sap from the stems of dandelions topically to the warts several times per day until they resolve, which may take several weeks.

Making Herb-Taking Fun

If you can get your child to take herbs without adding sweeteners—great! If not, use the best quality sweetener that you can. Maple syrup and brown rice syrup are preferable to honey. Or add a little dried

Honey can be dangerous for children under 1 year of age. It can contain *Clostridium botulinum,* a bacteria that very young digestive tracts may not have enough acidity to destroy. Good alternatives include maple syrup, rice syrup, and stevia.

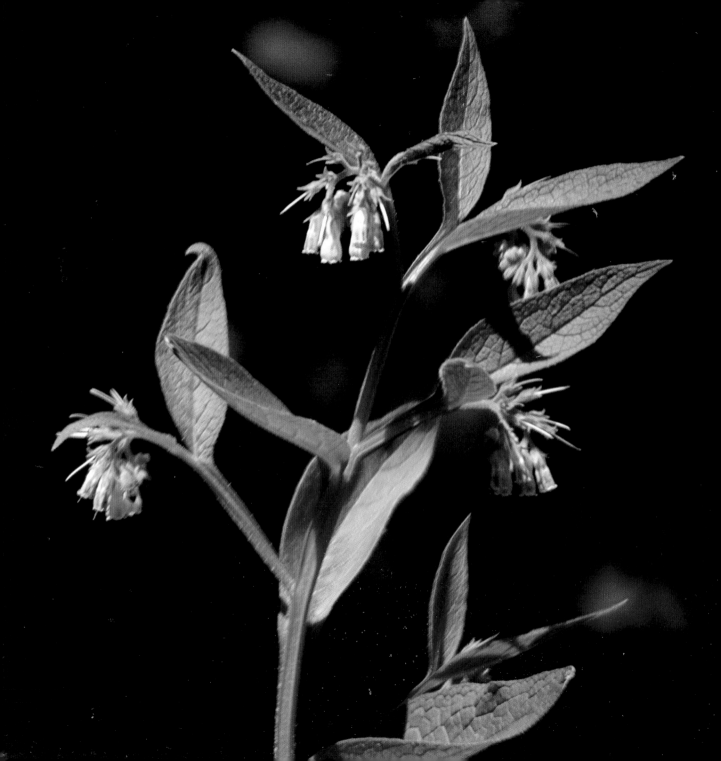

Chapter 12

Herbal First Aid

Supporting Self-Healing

When we apply a substance to the skin it is important to remember that the skin is filled with tiny capillaries, and things put on the skin are quickly absorbed into the systemic circulation. We therefore want to be as careful with whatever we put onto our skin as we are with whatever we put into our mouths. Many over-the-counter wound-healing preparations or muscle-pain relievers contain potentially harmful chemicals. Once in the bloodstream, they increase the burden on our liver and can impair cell health. Just as when taking medicine internally, when we apply therapeutics externally we want to first do no harm and then support the body's natural defenses. The herbs discussed in this chapter do just that.

They are nontoxic. They support the body's ability to fight off infection, they help to close open wounds, and they support the body in making new cells. And they are inexpensive, often free! What follows is a brief overview of how to use a few simple herbs to treat common household injuries. This is followed by a description of the benefits of these herbs for topical use and a solvent percentage (explained in Chapter 13) to help you make your own extract of the herb.

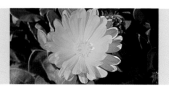

Calendula

CUTS

Use a calendula succus to wash any wound where the skin surface has been broken. For a superficial wound, place calendula tincture on a cotton ball and apply to the wound periodically. For a wound that you wish to keep covered, place calendula succus on the pad of a bandage and place it over the wound. Keep the wound covered with the bandage and calendula until new skin forms. If the wound is very painful, add St. John's wort tincture for pain relief.

BURNS

For first-degree burns, such as sunburns, apply nettles tincture and/or St. John's wort tincture to the affected area periodically until the pain has subsided. For kitchen burns, such as scalding or contact burns, immerse the affected part in cool water for up to 30 minutes. Then apply nettles and/or St. John's wort tinctures and allow to dry. If you chose to cover the burn, use a clean dry bandage. If the burn looks like it may become infected, apply a calendula succus. For chemical burns, flush the area with water immediately for 20 minutes and seek professional assistance. Burns are tolerated poorly by children under the age of five and by the elderly and are therefore of greater concern in these individuals.

BRUISES

Mix a few drops of St. John's wort tincture into some arnica oil and gently rub over the bruised area. This can be repeated until the discoloration and inflammation subside. Arnica can be irritating to a bleeding bruise; in this case apply the St. John's wort tincture alone to the bruise using a cotton swab.

BITES AND STINGS

Wash any bite first with calendula, then apply St. John's wort tincture to the wound periodically with a cotton ball or place the St John's wort on the pad of a bandage and cover the area of the bite. If the area of the bite is itchy and leaves a splotchy rash, consider applying nettles tincture.

A poultice of grated potato or mud will draw out the insect venom and soothe the inflammation. Clay is not exactly an herb. It is actually more fundamental than that—it is the Earth, itself. I generally use bentonite or green clay if I'm at home, which can also be found in most natural food stores. It is also possible to use clay found outdoors. When you do this, use fine-quality clay from several inches below the ground surface, if possible. Remove any rocks or course grains. If you are at home, place the clay in an oven long enough so that it is thoroughly warmed. Then, mix the clay with enough water to make a thick paste. Apply the clay evenly over the area to be treated with a the back of a spoon. Cover with gauze or some other kind of bandage. Leave the clay poultice on until the clay dries and pulls away from the skin. This is the most effective method for drawing out toxins or insect venom. If the purpose of the poultice is to soothe inflamed, irritated skin, keep the poultice moist with frequent applications of water over several hours.

STRAINS AND SPRAINS

Tradition tells us to use ice, elevation, rest, and the support of an ace bandage in the case of a recent strain or sprain. In addition, gently rub arnica oil onto the affected part, or mix arnica oil with St. John's wort tincture for added pain relief and decreased inflammation.

RASHES

A skin rash can be a representation of internal toxicity and simply addressing it with external applications will generally not bring about a lasting cure. See Chapter 4 on digestion and the role of the liver in skin health. However, herbs can also be used externally to soothe irritated skin while the systemic cause is being addressed, as in the Oatmeal Bath that follows. For intractable itching, use the neutral chamomile bath (Chapter 3).

Oatmeal Bath

MATERIALS

1 cup rolled oats
Stocking or sock

INSTRUCTIONS

Place the oats in a stocking or thin sock and knot it at the end to make an herbal bath bag. Begin filling the bath tub, or sink for infants, with hot water, letting the water from the faucet fall over the herbal bath bag. When the bath is approximately 1/3 full with the herbally infused water, continue to fill with cooler water. Monitor the temperature of the water to make it comfortable for bathing. Another technique is to fill the tub completely with hot water then let it cool to a comfortable temperature. The longer you have hot water running over the herbal bath bag, the stronger the herbal infusion will be. Squeeze the herbal bath bag periodically and watch the milky extract from the oats release into the water.

When the bath is a comfortable temperature, immerse your entire body in it. You can use the bath bag as a poultice to dab on affected areas.

After the bath, the oat bath bag can be stored in a zip-lock bag in the refrigerator for approximately 48 hours. During this time, remove the bag from the refrigerator and use as a poultice, applying it on irritated areas of the skin.

DOSE / TIMING / DURATION

This treatment can be used as often as necessary to relieve severe itching; however, spending too much time immersed in water may aggravate overly dry skin.

BENEFITS

Soothing to itchy irritated skin.

INDICATIONS

Itchy, irritated skin.

CAUTIONS

Water that is too hot can aggravate some skin conditions; let the water cool to a temperature slightly lower than you might usually use for a bath.

Alternating Hot and Cold

By alternating hot and cold, each application magnifies the healing effects of the previous one, thus adding up to more than they would have if done separately at widely spaced intervals. The combination is very effective for decongesting a congested area, relieving pain, and soothing irritated skin. See the Alternating Hot and Cold Sitz Bath here and the Hot Vinegar Pack in Chapter 13.

ALTERNATING HOT AND COLD SITZ BATH

An alternating hot and cold sitz bath is a powerful local treatment for rashes around the anus or genitals and for hemorrhoids. For a sitz bath a couple of inches of water are needed in separate containers—enough water cover the pelvic region. Immerse the pelvis in the tubs, alternating the hot bath (typically 3 minutes) with the cold bath (typically 30 seconds). Repeat three times, always starting with hot and finishing with cold.

For rashes, try using a hot herbal infusion of chamomile for the hot bath. For hemorrhoids add 3 tablespoons of witch hazel to both containers of water.

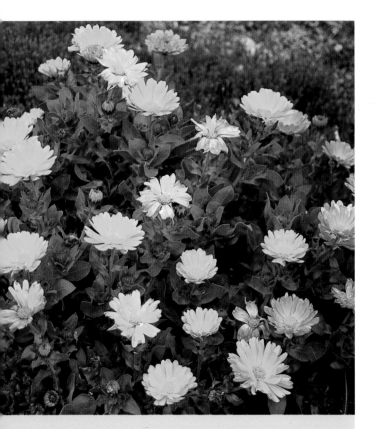

Calendula

Basic Herbal First Aid Kit

The herbal succuses, tinctures, and oils that follow make up a basic herbal first aid kit. They are wonderful to have on hand at home, in your car, or in your office so that, when the need arises, you don't have to go hunting for the appropriate tool. These can all be made quite simply when the herbs are in season; see Chapter 13 for instructions. For those of you who don't want to make your own, they are also available as a kit from The Art of Health, Inc.

There are, of course, many other herbs that can be grown in your garden or harvested from the wild to be used for first aid. The few herbs discussed here address our basic needs and therefore make a great start in building your own herbal first aid kit.

CALENDULA SUCCUS

This is the juice of the aerial parts of the calendula plant preserved with a small amount of alcohol. It cleans wounds, stops bleeding, and promotes tissue healing. Calendula is used externally on either open or closed wounds that are tender, red, swollen, and tending toward the formation of pus. It is used for inflamed skin conditions such as lacerations and burns (including sunburns) and other skin irritations such as diaper rash or eczema. When used early in the wound healing process, calendula can also prevent the formation of scar tissue.

ST. JOHN'S WORT TINCTURE

Known botanically as hypericum, St. John's wort tincture can be used externally on burns, puncture wounds, sores, boils, and insect and cat bites. It is specific for wounds with sharp, shooting pains, and wounds from sharp penetrating instruments. St. John's wort is also useful for bruises, neuralgias, and muscle strains, spasms, and aches. It has pain-relieving, anti-inflammatory, and tissue-healing properties. A few drops of St. John's wort tincture in water makes a pain-relieving mouthwash for gums that are sore from flossing or dental work (St. John's wort is safe to take internally, so do not be concerned if some is swallowed).

Solvent percentage for making an extract: 56–65%.

NETTLES TINCTURE

The botanical name for nettles is *Urtica urens.* Applied topically to a recent burn, nettles brings about rapid relief of pain and promotes tissue healing. Nettles is specific for burns that are stinging and/or itching and is also helpful on hives. For first- and second-degree burns, it can prevent the production of vesicles, inflammation, and scarring. It can also be applied to old burns to bring about more complete healing.

Solvent percentage for making an extract: 35–50%.

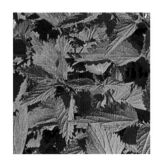

ARNICA OIL

Arnica is specific for bruises, strains, sprains, and discomfort from overexertion. It is best suited for blue and red swollen bruises when the wound is recent and the inflammation active. It is anti-inflammatory and antiseptic, it relieves pain from injuries, and promotes tissue regeneration. Arnica oil is **for external use only** and should not be used on bruises with bleeding because it can irritate exposed capillaries.

Solvent percentage for making an extract: 50–70%.

PLANTAIN

Plantain is very abundant because it uses the wind to pollinate. It is one of those plants that grows just about everywhere. I find it growing in my lawn, by the roadside, and through the cracks in sidewalks. Plantain has parallel-looking veins on its leaves that are reminiscent of the lily family. Be sure you have properly identified plantain before harvesting and using it because many members of the lily family are toxic. Plantain is often referred to as "nature's Band-Aid" because of its universal use in healing wounds. It can be used on irritated skin, itchy skin, bleeding wounds, inflammation, bee stings, and burns. Because it is safe to take internally, an effective use of plantain if you are away from home and wounded is to chew the leaves until they are well mashed and apply them topically to the wound as a poultice.

Plantain is also known to draw foreign objects, such as a sliver of glass or a splinter, out of the skin.

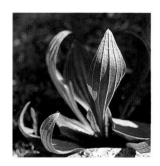

Its wound-healing properties include destroying a wide range of micro-organisms as well as stimulating the growth of new epithelium.

Solvent percentage for making an extract: 35–52%.

CHICKWEED

The botanical name for chickweed is *Stellaria media*. Chickweed is an incredibly common plant that grows as a weed all over the world. It is a highly nutritious green and makes a great addition to sal-

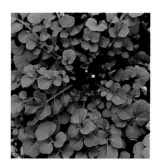

ads. Used externally, it is very useful when applied as a succus, oil, or poultice to treat skin irritations, inflammations and skin ulcers. It can also be used to draw out insect bites. It is astringent, cooling, and a demulcent. The best time to harvest chickweed is in the early spring when the greens are bright, but the plant is not yet flowering.

Solvent percentage for making an extract: 25–65%.

COMFREY

Comfrey contains allantoin, which encourages bone, cartilage, connective tissue, and muscle cells to grow. Comfrey works extremely quickly to heal wounds, so it should only be used on clean wounds so dirt is not trapped inside, which will cause infection.

Comfrey can also be applied to bone or muscle injuries, arthritic joints, or bruises. A comfrey poultice is highly indicated in cases of broken bones or

COMFREY POULTICE

To make a comfrey poultice, harvest comfrey leaves and/or root. Rinse and shake dry. Blend them with enough distilled water to create a thick mash. Place this mash on top of several layers of gauze and fold gauze to make an envelope to hold the comfrey. Apply this to the area to be treated, wrapping it with a roll of gauze, an ace bandage, or a bandanna to hold it in place.

An alternative method is to blend the comfrey with olive oil instead of water. The oil will help protect the skin from the potentially irritating "hairs" on the comfrey leaf.

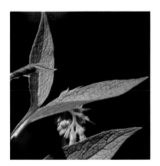

injured ligaments. The caution with comfrey is that it works extremely effectively and quickly, so make sure the broken bone has been set before using a comfrey poultice or the bone will be knit together improperly.

Solvent percentage for making an extract: 25–50%.

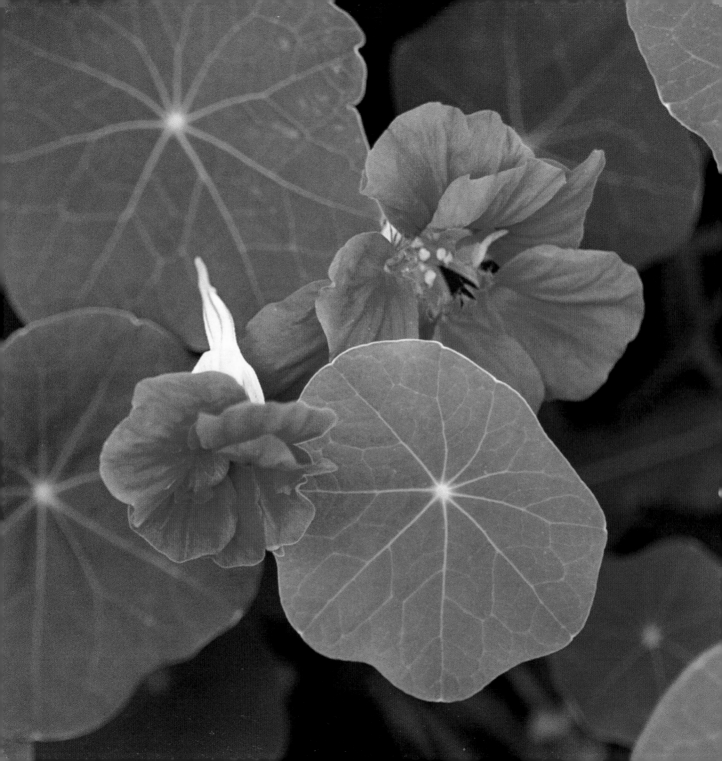

Chapter 13

From Garden to Pharmacy

Herb Garden: The Beginnings of an Herbal Pharmacy

A great way to get started in living with the herbs around you is to start a simple herb garden. Perhaps you have room for a garden in your yard or can plant herbs in and around other plants around your home. Herbs make great additions to perennial beds because they attract bees and butterflies, promoting pollination. If you don't have any garden space, you can start a garden in a planter box on your front stoop or kitchen window sill. With an herb garden of any size you can begin to observe the seasons in the cycles of

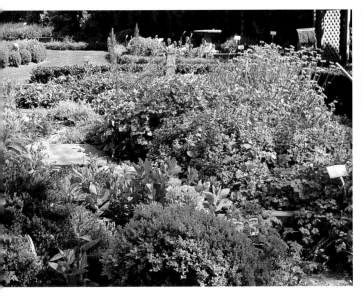

these because many of them spread prolifically. It is part of the nature of these great healing plants to make their healing properties available to us, and so they spread easily, grow lushly, become large, and die hard. Choose containers for some of these easily spreading herbs such as comfrey, mint, nettles. What follows is some information on a few easy-to-grow and very useful herbs to get you started.

COMFREY
(*Symphytum officinale*)

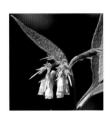

Comfrey is a perennial herb that grows 2–3 feet high and spreads 1–2 feet. You can begin harvesting the leaves in the spring and continue through the summer. Fall is the time to harvest the roots. Don't worry about killing comfrey when harvesting the roots—some will always be left behind and produce a hardy plant the following spring. Comfrey is one of those plants that is hard to eliminate once planted. It seems impossible to transplant comfrey without leaving a small piece of root in its original location, and that is all it takes for a new large and lush comfrey to grow the following season. So choose its location carefully. Comfrey is full of the constituent allantoin, which is

the plants, you will have some fresh herbs available to harvest when needed, and you will have herbs available to dry and store for later use.

You may already have a cooking herb garden. To start a garden for healing herbs, I suggest that you begin with the plants that grow easily and have little need for maintenance. Many herbs can be started by simply throwing some seeds on the ground in early spring and watching them grow. If you don't want a big wild garden, be careful how you plant some of famous as a wound healer. It knits wounds back together and is used to heal everything from fractures to bruises, insect bites, and minor cuts. An application of comfrey will close an open wound quickly, so make sure the wound is clean before applying comfrey.

Solvent percent: root 24–50%; leaf 50–65%.

MINTS

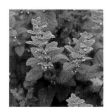

You can recognize a member of the mint family by its square branching stem. Common mints include peppermint (*Mentha piperita*), spearmint (*Mentha spicata*), and lemon balm (*Melissa officinalis*). Members of the mint family make great additions to a garden because they are easily grown, are highly aromatic, and have many medicinal uses. The leaves are the part of the plant used, and these are easily harvested and dried for teas. Collect the leaves on a hot, sunny day, preferably before the plant has flowered. These plants spread very easily by dropping seeds. Therefore if you want to contain their growth, plant your mint in a container on a porch or patio.

Solvent percent: 45–60%.

CALENDULA (*Calendula officinalis*)

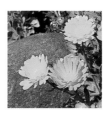

Calendula is easy to grow by simply sprinkling seeds on the ground and covering them slightly. The plant grows 1–2 feet high with a similar spread. The bright orange and yellow flowers that it produces are a delight to the eyes. Calendula is an annual and will bloom in early spring and continue throughout the summer. In milder climates, it may even bloom through the winter. Harvest the blossoms in the heat of the day and use them fresh to make a calendula succus—a fresh juice extraction of calendula preserved with a little alcohol to be used for wound healing. Dry the blossoms to store and use throughout the winter in tea. Calendula is also great for lymphatic stagnation—the succus or the tea could be taken internally for this use. The petals make a beautiful addition to salads.

Solvent percent: 50–80%.

NETTLES
(*Urtica urens*)

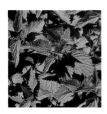

I grow nettles in my garden. Friends, having been stung by nettles in the wild, cautioned me against it. But I couldn't resist because nettles have so many very valuable everyday uses. Nettles are one of the most nutritious plants on the planet. They can be eaten as a cooked green, in much the same way as you eat cooked spinach. They can be juiced or used in tea, tincture, or a nutritive vinegar (see Chapter 6 on hormonal balance). They are extremely valuable in relieving the symptoms of allergies, they cleanse the kidneys, and topically they are a very important component of a first aid kit and used for burns that sting and itch (see Chapter 12). In the garden, nettles may grow up to 6 feet tall and with a spread of 2–3 feet. To keep the nettles from spreading their seeds and taking over your garden, cut them back and use the greens regularly before they flower and seed.

Solvent percent: 35–50%.

CHAMOMILE
(*Matricaria recutita* or *M. chamomilla*)

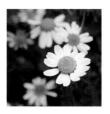

Chamomile is an annual that can be started easily from seed—either directly into the ground or by starting it inside and transplanting it outside after 8–10 weeks. Chamomile grows well in cool weather, so plant it in the early spring or fall. The plant grows 1–2 feet high and spreads only 4–15 inches. The blossoms can be used fresh or dried for a tea that will calm and soothe the nerves, digestion, promote sleep, and so on—the list of chamomile's benefits goes on and on. Chamomile is readily available in just about every supermarket, but I highly recommend growing some of your own. Homegrown chamomile is very special indeed.

Solvent percent: 45–65%.

ECHINACEA
(*Echinacea purpurea*)

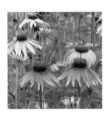

There are nine species of echinacea native to North America, but the one most commonly used medicinally is *Echinacea purpurea*. The flowers are a vibrant purple with orange centers. With this variety of echinacea, the entire plant can be used—roots, leaf, flower, and seeds. Echinacea will grow up to 4 feet high with a spread of 1–2 feet. Perennials such as echinacea take longer to establish themselves. The root of echinacea is ready for medicinal use after its third summer. The aerial parts, however, can be used the first or second years. If you are harvesting the aerial parts, cut at the point where the first healthy-looking leaves are growing when the flowers are just starting to open. The root is harvested in the fall. All parts of *Echinacea purpurea* can be used fresh to make a tincture or dried for use in teas.

Solvent percent: 45–75%.

ST. JOHN'S WORT
(*Hypericum perforatum*)

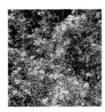

I have a large patch of St. John's wort in my herb garden. I started it by transplanting the volunteers that spontaneously appeared around our property. St. John's wort is another prolific reseeder, so your patch could potentially spread far and wide. I make tincture from my St. John's wort for my first aid kit (see Chapter 12), and to be used internally. It is also easy to dry and use in teas when the fresh herb is not available. St. John's wort is most potent in its bud form. Ideally it is harvested when the buds on the plant are numerous and the majority of them have not yet opened. If you pick a bud and rub it between your fingers, it will leave a strong red stain on your hands. This tells you that it is potent and ready to be harvested. The extract of St. John's wort that you make will have the deep red color.

Solvent percent: 56–65%.

Harvesting Herbs

Herbs are generally easy to grow, are hardy and not very susceptible to disease or pests. They are often quite adaptable to various soils and growing conditions. Now that you have planted some herbs and watched them grow, the next step is to harvest and use them.

Different parts of plants are harvested at certain times of year. You want to harvest from a plant at the time when it is concentrating its energy in the part of the plant that you will be using. For instance, St. John's wort flowers are most potent in bud form, so you want to harvest St. John's wort when the buds are plump but have not yet opened. In general, if you are harvesting flowers, do so just before they are fully expanded. Leaves should be harvested when the plant is young and the leaves fresh and vibrant looking. Usually leaves are harvested before the herb begins to develop its flower because at that point the energy of the plant begins to go into making the flower and seeds. Roots should generally not be harvested until the plant's third year. I think of gathering roots in the late fall when the aerial parts have died back and the attention of the plant has gone back underground, but before the ground itself gets too hard to dig. Fruits and berries are best picked ever so slightly before they ripen; seeds are best picked when they have fully ripened.

You may also, at times, have the opportunity to gather herbs that are growing in the wild (generally referred to as wild-crafting). In this circumstance, be careful to harvest in a way that will support continued abundance and natural beauty. Some guidelines for sustainable harvesting include gathering from places of abundance and only taking 1/4 of what is there at the most. Think about harvesting so that no one will be able to tell that you have been there.

After you have harvested or gathered your herbs the next step is to garble. To *garble* means to separate out the most desirable portions of the plant for medicine making. This includes removing any other plants that may be attached to the specimen, removing dead leaves, twigs, and, in some cases, excess stems. This can also be done after the plant has been dried, but I find it easier to do when the plant is fresh.

The next question is: Are you going to use the harvested plant immediately or do you want to save it for later use? The fresh plant consumed or used whole is the most potent form of herbal medicine. Examples of using herbs in this way include making a poultice out of a fresh herb for external application, harvesting fresh spring greens such as dandelions and using them in salads, and juicing dandelion and fresh nettles to add to other freshly juiced vegetables such as carrot, beet, and celery. A tea can also be made by infusing the fresh leaves or flowers of herbs such as chamomile or lemon balm.

If you want to capture the healing properties of the herb for later use, you can use the fresh herb to make an extract such as a tincture or a succus. If you are unable to process the herbs immediately, they can be placed in an airtight container and refrigerated for another day. However, the longer the time between the harvest and the time of processing, the less potent the extract will be. The herb is always most potent immediately after harvest.

There will be times when you want to harvest a plant because it is at its peak in potency, but not use it until later. Drying herbs is another way of saving herbs for later use. You can then use your dried herbs to make a tea, poultice, or an extract such as herbal oil, a tincture, or a glycerite. Simple instructions for drying and for making various kinds of extracts (tinctures, glycerites, vinegars, aqueous extracts, herbal oils, and succuses), salves, and poultices follow.

Drying Herbs

Generally herbs are best when dried rapidly. Herbs collected in the warm months can be air dried in a dark, well-ventilated room. In cooler, damp weather the room for drying should be heated to 70–100 degrees F. Ideally herbs should be dried on a mesh surface so that air can pass through them freely. You may want to hang a piece of cheesecloth over the herbs, but well above their surface to allow for air flow, to protect them from dust. Whole herbs or flowering tops can be tied loosely in small bundles and hung upside down—away from the wall is best, again to allow for the greatest amount of air flow. Dried herbs should hold their natural color and fragrance for about a year when properly stored in an airtight container in a cool, dark environment.

- For flowers: Flowers should be dried rapidly to retain their color, but never above 90 degrees F. Spread flower heads loosely over the drying surface stirring occasionally until they are dry.

- For roots: To facilitate the drying of roots, cut them into lengths no longer than 1/2 inch. They should also be stirred frequently during the drying process to prevent the growth of mold.

- For leaves: For thin leaves, a temperature of about 70 degrees F is appropriate; more succulent leaves require a temperature of about 90 degrees F. Separate the leaves from the stem and lay them on a drying surface until they are dry, stirring occasionally.

Making Your Own Medicine

Making medicines from herbs is actually quite simple. And, most important, the medicines that you make yourself are no less effective than those made in fancy factories and sold in stores. In fact, the ones you make yourself can be more potent for many reasons, most obviously because the ingredients you use may be fresher. Harvesting a small amount of herbs from your own garden and taking it directly to your kitchen for immediate processing into a tincture, vinegar, or poultice is probably much faster than the process of even the most conscientious manufacturer gathering a large quantity of a given plant, transporting it to the manufacturing facility, and processing it. The fresher the ingredients, the more potent the medicine. But there is another element to making your own medicines that is harder to describe. It has to do with the energy and intention that you put into making the medicine. Somehow the plant responds or you responded to the plant (most likely both are happening), and there is an increased flow between the plant and the person using it—this increased flow is a key factor in creating health.

In the herbal products industry right now, there is a movement toward *standardized* extracts—this means that a particular constituent of the plant (usually the one believed to be the active constituent) is standardized to a certain number of milligrams. This means that, if a given batch has less than the standard milligrams of this "marker" compound, then more is added. This turns herbal medicines into pharmaceuticals instead of using them in their natural forms. There are two problems with this:

- It is entirely possible that the "marker" compounds to which the product is being standardized is not actually the constituent of the herb that brings about the desired effects.

- The properties of a plant are never the result of one single compound—this is reductionist thinking. They are a result of the combination of plant constituents interacting in a very unique and sophisticated way. The myriad substances in each plant work together to create the effects of the plant in or on our bodies and also seem to act to balance one another out. This tends to make whole plant extractions safer, with fewer adverse reactions than a standardized drug made from the same herb.

To change the balance of constituents in a plant extract is arrogance on our part, and it is very much in keeping with the way we have altered the foods that we eat. Instead of eating food whole, the way that the Earth has provided them to us, we take out the parts that we don't like. When, as a result, the health of our population declined, we then started adding nutrients artificially to foods, fortifying them, to make up for the nutritious parts that we took out. Our health has not improved from these "advanced" techniques; it has declined. Chronic diseases of all kinds are steadily increasing. The best way to reverse this increase in disease is to return to the consumption of *whole* foods and medicines made from *whole* plants.

HERBAL EXTRACTS

A menstrum is a solvent used to extract the chemical constituents in herbs. Commonly used menstrums include water, alcohol, glycerine, and vinegar. The qualities we look for in a menstrum are its ability to dissolve, extract, and preserve the desired constituents of a herb. Different plant constituents are best extracted by different mediums, and for those that are best extracted by an alcohol/water menstrum, the percentage of alcohol of the menstrum is also important for getting the highest quality extract.

Choosing a Menstrum

There are many factors that go into choosing a menstrum. Alcohol is used most commonly because it extracts many plant constituents well, it kills most microbial activity, and it is an effective preservative. Alcohol extracts have the least potential for going bad and have a longer shelf life then many other extracts. Alcohol is an effective solvent for fats, resins, waxes, most alkaloids, glycosides, and some volatile oils. Alcohol does not dissolve gums, mucilage, albumins, or starches. It is generally estimated that extracts made in alcohol (tinctures) will be good for 2–5 years.

A nonalcohol alternative is a glycerite, an extract using a menstrum of vegetable glycerine or of vegetable glycerine and water. This is often used as an

Some plants containing resins: ginger, cayenne, and kava kava.

Some plants containing glycosides: St. John's wort, vitex, ginkgo, hawthorn, roses (wild and ornamental), cramp bark, licorice, gotu kola, and Siberian ginseng.

alternative to tinctures for children and others who wish to avoid alcohol. Glycerine is an effective menstrum for herbs containing tannins, alkaloids, bitter compounds, and sugars. It will not dissolve resins or fixed oils. Glycerine is the sweet, mucilaginous constituent of fats and oils and is **not** recommended for use with mucilaginous herbs such as comfrey or slippery elm. Glycerine has some antiseptic properties, but will not preserve herbs as well as alcohol. The shelf life of a glycerite is 1–3 years, depending on the water content of the herb used.

Herbal extracts can also be made using vinegar as a menstrum. Such an extract is formally called an acetum. Vinegar is the preferred menstrum for extracting alkaloids and will also extract vitamins and minerals. It is not effective in extracting plant acids. An acetum also has other benefits: It is nontoxic to the body (as opposed to alcohol, which is a stress on the liver), it helps to regulate the acid-alkaline balance of the body, and it is supportive of digestion. The shelf life of an acetum can vary from 6 months to several years.

Water is an effective solvent for starches, pectins, alkaloids, bitter compounds, saponins, glycosides, vitamins, proteins, tannins, mucilages, and sugars. Water alone will not preserve the extract. Water extracts such as infusions or decoctions should be used within 1 day or if refrigerated for 3–4 days.

Oils can also be used to make herbal extracts. Oils are effective solvents for wax (when heated), volatile oils, camphors, and some vitamins and minerals.

A succus uses fresh plant material that is ground up, sometimes with a small amount of added water, and then is expressed immediately and preserved with a small amount of alcohol. This is different than most other herbal extracts, in which the herb generally sits in the menstrum for a couple of weeks. I discuss calendula and plantain succuses in Chapter 12.

> **Some plants containing alkaloids:** goldenseal, Oregon grape, and comfrey.
>
> **Some plants containing tannins:** eucalyptus, green tea, cinnamon bark, cherry bark, and peppermint.

> **Some plants containing bitter compounds:** burdock, dandelion, catnip, gentian, goldenseal, hops, motherwort, and skullcap.
>
> **Some plants containing mucilage:** comfrey, oats, plantain, slippery elm, and borage.

Making Tinctures

A tincture is an herbal extract in a base of alcohol and water. The alcohol is used to extract the constituents from the plant, destroy microbes, and act as a preservative. When an alcohol tincture is well made, it can last 2–5 years.

Tinctures can be made either by the folk method, which is described here, or by the scientific method, which involves more precise measuring of the herb-to-menstrum ratio and therefore providing a measurement of the grams of herb per dose. On commercial products, this ratio is represented as 1:1, 1:2, or 1:5 herb-to-menstrum ratio.

To make an herbal extract via the folk method, place the chopped up dried or fresh herb in a clean jar with a tight (preferable non-metal) lid. Pour the desired menstrum over the herb, covering the herb and about 2 inches above it with menstrum. Make sure the jar you use is large enough that you will be able to shake the jar and the contents can move about freely. Cap the jar tightly. Give your herbal extract its first good shake and then store it out of direct sunlight. For the next 2 weeks, shake the mixture vigorously daily. After 2 weeks, use cheesecloth or a coffee filter over a strainer to capture the herb as you decant the liquid.

Some plants high in volatile oils: fennel, lemon balm, catnip, mints, cardamom, cinnamon, thyme, eucalyptus, lavender, and rosemary.

Store your tincture away from light and heat in a sealed container labeled with the contents and the date made.

Proof is the alcohol-to-water ratio of alcohol purchased in stores. By definition, proof is twice the percentage of alcohol in a liquid; for example, 80 proof vodka is 40% alcohol. Although there are specific percentages of alcohol that are recommended for different types of plants or plant constituents, 40% is a good middle range for extracting constituents from most herbs for home use. Therefore a simple way to make a home tincture is to use undiluted 80–90 proof vodka or to use a flavored brandy, which is often 40% alcohol, as your menstrum. A more economical menstrum is 180 proof grain alcohol, diluted 50% grain alcohol to 50% water. This will be less expensive, but also less palatable. Because fresh herbs have much higher water content than dried, consider using a much higher alcohol-content menstrum for fresh herbs, such as 90% alcohol, while using a 40–60% alcohol menstrum for dried herbs.

Making Glycerites

For children and those who do not tolerate alcohol, herbs can be extracted in glycerine. Glycerine is sweet to the taste, which makes many herbs more palatable. As mentioned earlier, the disadvantage of glycerine is that it does not extract many plant constituents as well as alcohol. For this reason, many companies that prepare herbal products today do the extraction in alcohol, then distill off the alcohol and add glycerine as a preserving and flavoring base. But for home purposes, extracting in glycerine or in glycerine and water is completely adequate.

When preparing a menstrum out of glycerine, two parts glycerine to one part water is generally used. Use at least 60% glycerine when making a glycerite to insure adequate preservation of the extract. Be sure to use vegetable-based glycerin in your herbal preparations rather than an animal- or petroleum-based one.

A glycerite should last 1–3 years; the more water in the plant—that is, the fresher the plant—the shorter the shelf life, so a glycerite made from a dried plant will have a longer shelf life. To help preserve a glycerite and extend its shelf life you can add essential oils, vitamin C, or store it in the refrigerator.

You can make a glycerite in much the same way as a tincture, except that the menstrum is either 100% pure vegetable glycerine (for fresh herbs) or a mixture of glycerine and water, for example, 75% glycerine to 25% water (for dried herbs). Place the dried or fresh herb in a blender and cover it with the menstrum. Blend well and place the mixture in a glass jar. Let the combination sit for 2 weeks, shaking it vigorously twice daily. Strain out and press the herb, and store the glycerite in an amber-colored bottle; if you are using a clear glass jar, then store it out of direct light. A recipe for hawthorn glycerite can be found in the Chapter 9; there are also glycerites for children mentioned in Chapter 11.

Making Herbal Vinegars

Vinegar is technically an acid liquid made from wine, cider, or beer by a process of fermentation. It is believed that it is the fermenting process that gives the vinegar its healing capacities and the dramatic increase in nutrients from its original source.

Herbal vinegars (acetums) have been used for thousands of years. Organic apple cider vinegar is the best choice to make an herbal extract with vinegar. Good quality vinegar comes from the best quality apples. That means apples that have been grown without pesticides on fertile rich soil and then processed with care—not exposed to excess heat and certainly not pasteurized. As mentioned earlier, vinegars are effective in extracting alkaloids, vitamins, and minerals. That's why the herbal vinegars recommended in this book are primarily nutritive tonics, a way of adding vitamins and minerals directly from plants to the diet.

Apple cider vinegar is one of those substances that have been proclaimed cure-alls. It can be taken internally or applied externally for numerous situations: it not only can be used to restore balance when we become ill, but it is an excellent tool for promoting and sustaining wellness. Apple cider vinegar is full of vitamins and minerals, (B vitamins, calcium, boron, manganese, silicon, and magnesium), essential amino acids, and enzymes. It is also high in complex carbohydrates and dietary fiber. Applied externally to the skin, apple cider vinegar helps normalize the skin's pH because it has a pH that is very close to that of healthy skin.

Some examples of herbal vinegars and their uses are given here. See also the Digestive Tonic and Super Salad Dressing in Chapter 4.

An herbal vinegar is made using the same process as is used to make a tincture by the folk method, but instead of an alcohol and water menstrum, an apple cider vinegar menstrum is used. Place the fresh or dried herb into a jar and cover it with apple cider vinegar. Let the mixture cure for 6 weeks, and then strain out the herb. The herbal vinegar is then ready

MORE BENEFITS OF APPLE CIDER VINEGAR

- Apple cider vinegar is both antiseptic and antibiotic; it binds cholesterol and draws it out of the body. Decreasing cholesterol in the body reduces risks of cardiovascular disease.

- In cooking it can be added to a pot of cooking beans to make them more easily digestible.

- To ease a sore throat, gargle with 1 tablespoon apple cider vinegar in a cup of warm water.

SOME HERBAL VINEGARS AND THEIR USES

Dandelion vinegar is a wonderful way to include this deeply supportive herb into the diet. Dandelion vinegar can be used as a salad dressing or mixed with warm water and drunk before meals. This is an easy way to benefit from dandelion's immune and digestive support, liver cleansing, and diuretic properties.

Peppermint or spearmint vinegar settles and calms the digestive tract. Add a couple of teaspoons of peppermint vinegar to a glass of water to ease stomach cramps, diarrhea, or gas and bloating. A teaspoon of honey can be added to make a delicious-tasting remedy for indigestion.

Eucalyptus vinegar is vinegar that has extracted the aromatic oil of eucalyptus. Adding some of this vinegar to an herbal steam inhalation (see Chapter 8) will help clear a stuffy head or clogged respiratory system.

NASTURTIUM VINEGAR

1 quart Nasturtium flowers
2 cloves Garlic
1 quart apple cider vinegar

Combine the ingredients and age 6 weeks. Strain out the herbs and use. Nasturtiums are good for breaking up congestion and expectorating mucus in the respiratory passageways. Take 1/2 teaspoon in a small amount of warm water up to 6 times per day during an acute cold with congestion.

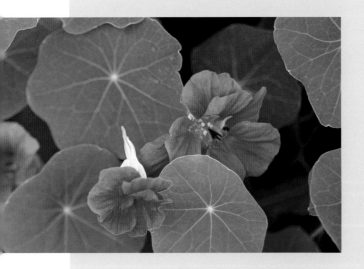

GARLIC VINEGAR

Place the peeled cloves of an entire bulb of garlic in a quart of apple cider vinegar and allow to sit for 2 weeks. Strain out and discard the garlic.

Add this vinegar to any dish for which the flavor of garlic is indicated. Add it to flax oil for a health-enhancing salad dressing.

HOT VINEGAR PACK

The hot vinegar pack is an effective pain-relieving therapy.

Make a mixture of 50% herbal vinegar and 50% water. Heat the mixture until steaming hot. Soak a towel in the vinegar mixture. Use heavy kitchen gloves to wring out the hot towel, and then shake it to cool it to a temperature that is comfortable to the body. Apply the towel to the desired area of the body. Leave it on for 5 minutes. Remove the vinegar-soaked towel, wring out a towel soaked in cold water, and apply it for 5 minutes, covered with wool. Repeat three times. Be sure to resoak the towel in the hot vinegar solution with each hot application and to finish with the cold towel.

to use. Store in a tightly sealed bottle at room temperature.

When herb vinegars are used for medicinal purposes, 1–3 teaspoons in a glass of water are generally used. But these herbal vinegars also can be used to promote wellness when used as salad dressings or to flavor meat or vegetable dishes.

Making Aqueous Extracts

When water is the menstrum used to make an herbal extract we have an aqueous extract. There are primarily two aqueous extracts—infusions and decoctions. Water is said to be the "universal solvent"; it has the most extensive range of all the liquid solvents. Thus, aqueous extracts are probably the most important of all herbal medicines. The downside, however, of aqueous extracts is that water does not act as a preservative, so the extract will only last about 24 hours at room temperature and 3–4 days refrigerated. Aqueous extracts contain the most active constituents of all liquid extracts, but have the shortest shelf life.

Infusion is the process used for most tea making. The process of infusion is generally used for the arial parts of plants such as flowers and leaves. Use 1 heaping teaspoon of herbs for each cup of water. Warm the steeping container first. The herb is placed in the empty steeping container and then just boiled water is added. Cover, and let sit from 5 to 15 minutes. Strain out the herb, and the aqueous extract is ready for use. There are many tools available for infusing herbs for drinking as tea: wire mesh balls, teaspoon infusers, French presses, and so on.

Decoction is used for harder plant parts, such as roots, barks and seeds, and dried berries. Use 1 tablespoon of herb for every cup of water. Place the herb and cold water in a sauce pan, turn on the heat, and bring the water to a boil. Cover the pan with a well-fitting lid and simmer for 15 minutes. Remove the pan from the burner and let the liquid steep another 10 minutes. Strain out the herb and use the decoction.

Once you have made an aqueous extract, either by infusion or decoction, the extract can be taken internally as a tea, applied to the body as a compress, or used as a soak for part or all of the body. The use of an aqueous extract as a compress or soak is part of hydrotherapy (see later in this chapter). There are examples of aqueous extractions throughout the book; see the recipes for teas and baths.

Herbal Oils

There are two kinds of herbal oils: extractions made with fixed oils and essential oils. Fixed oils are extracted from fruits, nuts and seeds, such as avocados, olives, castor beans, almonds, or grape seeds. We can then use this oil to create an herbal oil—an herbal extract using a fixed oil as the menstrum. Making an herbal oil is similar to making a tincture. The herb should be placed in the bottom of a glass jar and covered with about 2 inches of the fixed oil. If you are using leaves, they should be finely chopped; if you are using berries or flower buds, you may keep them whole. Let the oil and herb mixture sit for 2 weeks. If you are using a fresh herb, you must open the jar and wipe off any condensation daily so it will not grow mold. It is easier to use dried herbs for making herbal oils.

Here are some examples of common fixed oils.

- Almond oil is the oil that is most commonly used for massage oils. It is light and has little to no odor, and it is the least expensive of the lighter oils.

- Grape seed oil is a more expensive, but highly therapeutic oil. Grape seed oil has anti-oxidant properties and is light, and odorless, and highly emollient.

- Olive oil is the oil most commonly used as a solvent when the finished herbal oil is to be used as a food. Olive oil is highly nutritious, is stable when exposed to heat, and has a delicious flavor.

- Sesame oil is used as a base for many Ayurvedic therapies. Sesame herbal oils can be used both internally and externally. Sesame oil itself is warming and easily penetrates and nourishes the skin when used topically.

- Castor oil is my favorite oil for external use. Castor oil has many healing properties in its own right. It is anti-inflammatory, pain relieving, cleansing, able to dissolve abnormal tissue growths, stimulating to the immune system, and balancing to the nervous system (see the Castor Oil Pack Treatment in Chapter 10). Castor oil works very well when mixed with other herbal oils such as a St. John's wort, comfrey, or oil of arnica flowers.

You can also use fixed oils and herbs to make poultices (e.g., the olive oil and comfrey poultice in Chapter 12). For some uses of arnica oil, see Chapter 12 (the section on this oil, and also under bruises and strains and sprains).

The second kind of herbal oil is the essential oils. These are quite different. Essential oils are highly concentrated volatile oils taken directly from a plant via a distillation process. These oils are highly aromatic and evaporate quickly. Essential oils are therapeutic when inhaled (aromatherapy) and when absorbed through the skin. In aromatherapy, because essential oils are highly aromatic and are composed of very small molecules, they quickly dissolve into the mucus lining of the nasal passages where they transmit signals to the main olfactory nerves. This information is carried quickly to the brain, which triggers the release of hormones from the hypothalamus. Used topically, the small size of the essential oil molecules also makes them easily absorbed through the skin. Evidence that they are absorbed into the bloodstream comes from the presence of the oils in perspiration, feces, urine, and breath after topical applications. Applying essential oils (they should **always** be diluted, except for lavender essential oil) is a way of getting the wonderful healing plant constituents right to the area that needs help, so the response is faster and stronger. Essential oils can be blended to work synergistically; however, as a beginner you should use only one oil at a time. Because the oils do affect one another, blending incompatible essential oils together will interfere with their function.

The process of making an essential oil is quite intricate and not easy to do at home. It is best to buy high-quality essential oils and keep them on hand for home use. Essential oils come in very small bottles that seem expensive; the bottles are expensive because many pounds of the plant are used to make a single ounce of essential oil, and they are so highly concentrated only a very small amount is used—often only a few drops at a time. To make essential oils less expensive, some companies may dilute them with fixed oils. When purchasing essential oils look for pure, undiluted essential oils.

Castor oil is thick and beautifully healing to dried cracked skin. I recently had a very painful crack in my heel that made it extremely difficult for my foot to bear weight. I put castor oil on a large Band-Aid and put it over the heel crack. I covered the Band-Aid with a sock and went to bed. In the morning, the heel was much less painful and I could put weight on the heel and walk almost completely normally. I continued to use the castor oil Band-Aid under my sock day and night. Within 3 days, the crack was completely healed.

GENERAL APPLICATIONS OF ESSENTIAL OILS

- In the bath, use 6–8 drops per bath or perhaps 1/2 as much with oils that can be irritating to the skin such as peppermint, lemon, or thyme.

- For compresses use 6 drops of essential oil in a bowl of hot or cold water.

- For massage, add up to 18 drops of essential oil for each ounce of fixed oil. This is a suggested amount. Because every individual has a different sensitivity to essential oils, as with all therapeutics, you may find this too strong for you and wish to use less. No more than 9 drops should be used for children or those with sensitive skin.

- For steam inhalations, add 3–5 drops of essential oil to a bowl of hot water.

PRECAUTIONS FOR ESSENTIAL OILS

- Keep in mind the strength of pure essential oils. One teaspoon of some essential oils taken internally could be lethal.

- Many essential oils are contraindicated during pregnancy. If you are pregnant, consult a Naturopathic healthcare practitioner before using essential oils other than lavender.

- If you have a chronic health condition (such as high blood pressure, epilepsy, or diabetes), consult a Naturopathic physician or healthcare practitioner familiar with the use of essential oils before using essential oils other than lavender, peppermint, and eucalyptus as described in this book.

Making Succuses

A succus is a fresh plant extract that is preserved with a small amount of alcohol. The total alcohol content is 10–15%, as opposed to the 45–85% alcohol found in most tinctures. A succus is further distinguished from a tincture in the way it is made. To make a tincture, the menstrum and herb are mixed together and then left for an extended period of time. The process of making a succus is started and finished in 1 day.

To make a succus, place the fresh plant in a blender or food processor. If the plant is high in its water content, you may not need to add water. If the plant is drier and does not mash well, add a small amount of water gradually. When the herb is well macerated, press the liquid portion out. This can be accomplished by pouring the maceration through cheesecloth, and then squeezing the cheesecloth well, expressing as much of the liquid as possible. This liquid is the succus; the remaining herb can be sprinkled over your garden bed as fertilizer. To preserve the succus, add a small amount of alcohol to equal at least 10%. See Chapter 12 for uses for succuses of calendula and plantain.

MAKING SALVES AND CREAMS

A salve is a semi-hardened herbal oil that melts when applied to the skin. Beeswax is used to provide firmness and oil supports the absorption of the healing properties of the herbs by the skin. Salves are a convenient way of applying herbs to wounds or to dry or eczematous skin.

To make a salve, you need 2 cups of an herbal oil such as calendula, plantain, chickweed, comfrey, or St. John's wort or a combination of these and 1-1/2 ounces of shredded beeswax (use a cheese grater or chop it finely with a knife). Heat the herbal oil in the top of a double boiler with water in the bottom over low heat. Slowly add the beeswax until a desirable consistency is obtained. To test the consistency, dip a chilled metal spoon (one that has been placed in the freezer for a few minutes) into the mixture of herbal oil and wax. If a cloudy coating appears shortly after dipping, then your consistency is right. Take the oil off the heat. If you wish to add essential oils to your salve, you can do so now (for example, for these herbs you might add 1/2 teaspoon lavender essential oil). Pour the salve into clean glass or plastic containers and let sit uncovered or lightly covered with a paper towel to keep debris out. Let it cool and harden before covering with a lid.

You may want to add 1–2 tablespoons of vitamin E oil and/or vitamin A oil to the salve before pouring it into the container to solidify. These are not only nourishing to the skin, but will also act to preserve the salve—to help keep it from going rancid. The shelf life of a salve is dependent on the ingredients. Smelling the salve will clearly indicate whether it has gone rancid. The salve can be stored at room temperature; refrigerate it to prolong its freshness.

To turn your salve into an herbal cream, you need an amount of water equal to the amount of oil, in this case 2 cups. The water can be distilled water, an herbal tea, or rose or lavender water. In a separate pot from the oil and beeswax mixture, heat the water (or tea) to the same temperature as the oil mixture. (Use a thermometer to make sure the water and the oil and beeswax mixture are truly at identical temperatures; I have had disastrous results when they were not!) Pour your water mixture into a blender and turn it on high. Very slowly add the oil and beeswax mixture as the blender is blending. When the cream looks thick, turn the blender off. The cream will continue to thicken as it cools. Jars of cream will last longest if refrigerated.

MAKING POULTICES

A poultice is an application of a plant in its whole form, as opposed to the application of an aqueous extract, succus, or oil of the plant. A poultice can be made from either fresh or dried plants—fresh is always better if it is available. The application of a poultice functions to soothe irritated skin, relieve pain, reduce inflammation, heal wounds, promote circulation, warm and relax muscles, and draw out toxins or foreign particles. Many herbs can be used as poultices. Some of my favorites are comfrey and plantain (see Chapter 12).

To make a poultice, blend the herb into a paste, using a blender or food processor and adding water if necessary. The desired consistency is wet, but not runny. Place the herbal paste directly on the skin and cover with gauze or some other cloth to secure the poultice in place. Before electricity, the method for making a poultice was to chew the leaves into a paste and place it over the wound. This method is especially indicated for herbs containing mucilage such as plantain or comfrey. These plants are quite abundant and thus are easy to find when we are away from home and may have need to tend to a wound. See the description of plantain as a poultice in Chapter 12.

Herbs and Hydrotherapy

Hydrotherapy, as the name implies, is the use of water either externally or internally in the treatment of disease or the promotion of health. It might, however, be more accurately described as thermotherapy because generally hydrotherapy treatments are about the application of hot and cold. Water just happens to be a wonderful medium with which to apply hot and cold.

Why water? Water is a wonderful conductor of heat; it carries heat to and from the body 25 times faster than air does. Its fluidity makes it easy to apply—it bends around a body part with perfect ease, making contact with every contour of the body. Water is readily available and is inexpensive. Water is also an easy way to extract healing constituents from herbs and apply them to the body.

I mentioned earlier that Naturopathic medicine focuses on supporting the body's ability to heal itself, not on overwhelming the body or doing the work for it. Hydrotherapy is a great example of this principle. Hydrotherapy techniques, through the application of hot and cold, affect the circulation to take advantage of its life-supportive properties. The circulation of blood is the way that every cell in our body receives the nutrition that it needs to function. Circulation is also the way that the body rids itself of wastes—substances that the body either cannot use at all or has more than enough of. A lack of nutrition or the buildup of wastes leads to disease—lack of nutrition weakens the body's ability to heal itself and the buildup of wastes is a stress on the body.

Hydrotherapy techniques both improve blood flow to an area in need of healing and optimize the quality of the blood; they make sure that the blood is carrying the appropriate nutrients as it circulates through the body. Optimizing blood flow to an area may mean increasing or decreasing circulation, depending on the circumstances. To improve the quality of blood, we can use hydrotherapy techniques to enhance blood flow through the organs of elimination such as the skin, liver, kidneys, and bowels. This helps to detoxify the blood, improving its quality. Hydrotherapy techniques tonify the digestive organs and improve the nutrition received by the blood, also improving its quality.

Hydrotherapy treatments appear throughout the book, including the Warming Sock Treatment (Chapter 3), the Constitutional Hydrotherapy Treatment (Chapters 4 and 11), several herbal baths (Chapters 2, 3, 7, 8, 11, and 12), the Herbal Steam Inhalation (Chapter 8), and the Hot Foot Bath (Chapter 5).

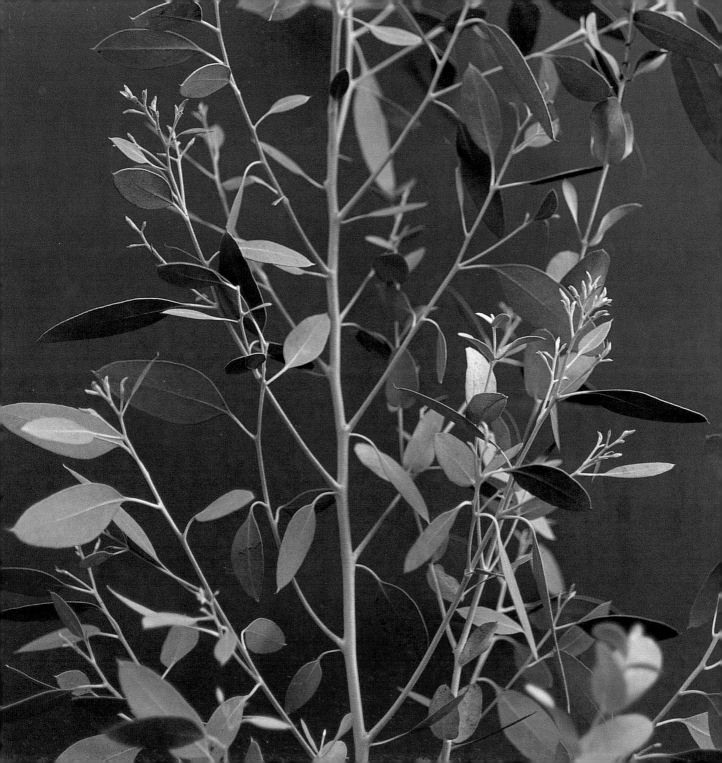

Epilogue

This book shares my understanding of health and wellness, which stems from the idea that humans are dynamic organisms constantly interacting with their environment and using this exchange to grow and develop and to *be* at an optimal level. In this book, I have illustrated that in this constant exchange with our environment there is the potential to overwhelm the body's homeostatic mechanisms and create imbalance or disease. I have described that part of maintaining a dynamic balance as we grow and constantly change is to live in accordance with our natural surroundings and that growing, harvesting, and consuming herbs as food and medicine is one way to accomplish this. Finally, I have discussed how, when we ignore or try to override the body's needs, we become out of balance and ill. We can use herbs first to help us observe the cycles in nature acting as a model for us, to help us maintain balance as we constantly experiment with different ways of exchanging with our environment (in other words, living), and to help us reclaim health when we have gone too far out of balance and we find ourselves ill in some way.

I intend this book to be a guide to beginning to live with the plants that naturally grow around you and using them to help you find vibrant health. Vibrant health is not found by balancing our body with pharmaceuticals—it is found when we unleash the wellness within us. There is no magic pill that will do this for us. Finding a vibrant state of health and well-being is a process, a very personal process that no one or thing—no doctor, no healer, no medicine—can do for us. It is something that unfolds as we take personal responsibility for our state of health and well-being. There are many things that each of us may find that will aid us in this process: spending time in nature; using movement therapies such as yoga, Qi gong, and Tai chi; practicing meditation; journal or poetry writing; using bodywork therapies; and more. This book is about the gift of herbs in helping us to find this vibrant state of health and well-being that is available to all of us.

Resources

Many of the teas described in this book, as well as kits for some of the therapies described, are available through The Art of Health, Inc., founded by Laura Washington, N.D. They are can be found at www.art-health.com or by phone at 800-816-8174.

To find a Naturopathic physician near you, contact one of the two accredited Naturopathic colleges. Both schools have a directory of practitioners on their websites.

Bastyr University
Kenmore, WA
425-823-1300
www.bastyr.edu

National College of Naturopathic Medicine
Portland, OR
503-499-4343
www.ncnm.edu

Bibliography

Boyle, Wade, and Andre Saine. *Lectures in Naturopathic Hydrotherapy*. Buckeye Naturopathic Press, 1988.

Brinker, Francis. *Herb Contraindications and Drug Interactions*, 2nd ed. Eclectic Medical Publications, 1998.

Brooke, Elisabeth. *Herbal Therapy for Women*. Thorsons, 1992.

Chetanananda, Swami. *Dynamic Stillness, Part One: The Practice of Trika Yoga*. Rudra Press, 1973.

Chetanananda, Swami. *Dynamic Stillness, Part Two: The Fulfillment of Trika Yoga*. Rudra Press, 1973.

Fallon, Sally, with Mary G. Enig. *Nourishing Traditions: The Cookbook That Challenges Politically Correct Nutrition and the Diet Dictocrats*, 2nd ed. New Trends Publishing, 1999.

Fischer-Rizzi, Susanne. *Medicine of the Earth: Legends, Recipes, Remedies, and Cultivation of Healing Plants*. Rudra Press, 1996.

Green, James. *The Herbal Medicine-Maker's Handbook*, 4th ed. Wildlife & Green Publications, 1990.

Guyton, Arthur C. *Textbook of Medical Physiology*, 8th ed. W. B. Saunders, 1991.

Lebot, Vincent, Mark Merlin, and Lamont Lindstrom. *Kava the Pacific Elixir: The Definitive Guide to Its Ethnobotany, History, and Chemistry*. Healing Arts Press, 1992.

Lust, John. *The Herb Book*. Bantam Books, 1987.

Mars, Brigitte. *Dandelion Medicine: Remedies to Detoxify, Nourish, Stimulate*. Storey Books, 1999.

McGarey, William A. *The Oil That Heals: A Physician's Successes with Castor Oil Treatments*. ARE Press, 1993.

Nuzzi, Debra. *Herbal Preparations and Natural Therapies: Creating and Using a Home Herbal Medicine Chest*. Morningstar Publications, 1989.

Sherman, John A. *The Complete Botanical Prescriber*. John A. Sherman, 1993.

Sturdivant, Lee, and Tim Blakley. *The Bootstrap Guide to Medicinal Herbs in the Garden, Field & Marketplace*. San Juan Naturals, 1999.

Thacker, Emily. *The Vinegar Book*, 12th ed. Tresco Publishers, 1996.

Thrash, Agatha, and Calvin Thrash. *Home Remedies: Hydrotherapy, Massage, Charcoal and Other Simple Treatments*. Thrash Publications, 1981.

Tilgner, Sharol. *Medicine from the Heart of the Earth*. Wise Acres Press, 1999.

Tisserand, Robert, and Tony Balacs (eds.). *Essential Oil Safety: A Guide for Health Care Professionals*. Churchill Livingstone, 1995.

Wood, Mathew. *The Book of Herbal Wisdom: Using Plants as Medicines*. North Atlantic Books, 1997.

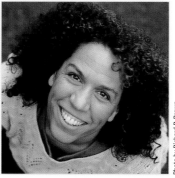

Photo by Richard P. Brown

About the Author

Laura Washington is a Naturopathic physician licensed and practicing in the state of Oregon. She received her doctor of naturopathic medicine from the National College of Naturopathic Medicine (NCNM) in Portland in 1998. She has served as adjunct faculty at NCNM and Lewis & Clark College. She is founder of The Art of Health, Inc., a company providing herbal teas and other therapeutic tools such as warming sock and herbal first aid kits. These and the other The Art of Health, Inc., products are designed to nourish and support the body's self healing mechanism.

As a physician and wellness educator, she enjoys working with people in the process of discovering health and wellness in a truly holistic manner. Dr. Washington uses traditional Naturopathic treatment modalities such as homeopathy, botanical medicine, nutrition, hydrotherapy, and various bodywork techniques. In addition to these approaches, she also uses Hatha Yoga, which she has taught extensively to groups and individuals for over 12 years.

Subject Index

Note: For specific herbs, see the Herb Index.

abdominal pain, 55
acetums, *see* vinegars, herbal
acne, 57, 58, 89
acupressure, 126
adaptogens, 33
addictions, eliminating, 33, 117-19, 120-23
   herbal teas, 33, 47, 119, 120
   other treatments, 119, 122, 123
AIDS, 20, 70
alcohol in tinctures, 157, 159
alcohol use, 53, 87, 88, 120
alkaloid herbs, 158
allantoin, 147, 150
allergies, 55, 62, 99, 100, 127, 131
   herbal teas, 98, 99
   herb cautions, 26, 48, 50, 103, 120
   other treatments, 98, 133, 152
Allergy Clearing Detox Tea™, 98, 99, 100
almond oil, 127, 164
alterative herbs, 46, 52, 131
Alternating Hot and Cold Sitz Bath, 143
alternating hot/cold treatments, 133, 143, 162
anemia, 43, 55
angina, 113
anti-inflammatory herbs, 27, 50, 100, 145, 164
anti-microbial herbs, 100, 103, 106, 146
antispasmodic herbs, 21, 50, 100, 103, 106, 130
anxiety, 20, 31, 41, 55
   herbal teas, 22, 23, 35, 82
   hydrotherapy, 38, 134, 135
apple cider vinegar, 46, 55, 160-61
   cautions, 54
   Hot Vinegar Pack, 143, 162
   see also vinegars, herbal
aqueous extracts, 155, 158, 163
   see also hydrotherapy, herbal; teas, herbal
aromatherapy, 164
arteriosclerosis, 113, 115
arthritis, 55, 57, 59

The Art of Health, Inc., 114, 144, 171
asthma, 20, 50, 55, 95, 100
   herbal teas, 113
   other treatments, 106
atherosclerosis, 109, 115
autoimmune disease, 53, 70
Ayurvedic medicine, 57

Bath and Sweat Treatment, 72, 104-5
bentonite, 141
berberine, 64
bites/stings, 141, 145, 146, 147, 151
bitter compounds, 158
bloating, 20, 44, 47
   herbal teas, 48, 82
   hydrotherapy, 49-50, 128-29
blood cleansing herbs, 13, 21, 22
blood thinning herbs, 110
blood-vessel dilating herbs, 110
boils, 58
bone fractures, 147, 151
brain function, 90, 91, 92
breathing therapy, 28, 72, 96
bronchitis, 100
   herbal teas, 97, 107
   hydrotherapy, 36-37, 72, 104-5
   other treatments, 56, 70, 106
bruises, 140, 145, 147, 151
burns, 140, 145, 146, 152

caffeine use
   eliminating, 33, 53, 117, 119, 120, 122
   results of, 33, 53, 63, 80, 87, 88, 127
Calming Herbal Baths, 25, 87, 134, 135
cancer, 18, 20, 47, 61-62, 63
carbuncles, 58
cardiovascular function, 18, 20, 21, 95, 109-11, 113
   glycerites, 112, 114
   herbal teas, 113, 114, 115
   hydrotherapy, 37, 38, 169
   other treatments, 13, 110-11, 114-15

cardiovascular problems
   heart failure, congestive, 89, 109, 113
   heart palpitations, 22, 114
   valvular murmur/regurgitation, 113
carminative herbs, 47-48
castor oil, 127, 164
Castor Oil Pack Treatment, 119, 122, 123, 164
children, treatment of, 125-27, 130-31, 133-37
   dosage, 135
   glycerites, 131, 133, 158, 160
   herbal teas, 130, 131
   hydrotherapy, 127, 128-29, 133, 134, 135
   nursing mother's diet, 127
   other treatments, 132, 133
   sweeteners, 133, 137
cholesterol, high, 113
claudication, intermittent, 113, 115
Clear Skin Tea, 58
colds, 18, 64, 66
   herbal teas, 70, 98, 99
   hydrotherapy, 36-37, 49-50, 72, 128-29
   other treatments, 69, 132
Comfrey Poultice, 147, 164
concentration, lack of, 20, 41, 44
congestion
   herbal teas, 98, 99
   hydrotherapy, 36-37, 38, 72, 74, 143
   other treatments, 98-99, 133
constipation, 18, 20, 44, 47, 51-52, 55, 123, 131
   in children, 131
   treatments, 52, 123, 131
Constitutional Hydrotherapy Treatments, 49-50, 127, 128-29, 169
Cough and Cold Syrup for Children, 106, 132, 133
coughs, 56, 97, 100, 106, 132
coumarin, 81
creams, 168

Cup of Sunshine Tea™, 92

dandelion vinegar, 161
decoctions, 21, 23, 33-34, 88, 158, 163
    see also aqueous extracts; teas, herbal
depression, 20, 41, 55, 77, 87, 88-89
    herbal teas, 82, 89, 92
    hydrotherapy, 25-26, 134, 135
detoxification, 66, 72, 96
    eliminating addictions, 121-22, 123
    herbal teas, 33, 52, 59, 89, 97-100,
        121-22, 131
    hydrotherapy, 72, 104-5, 169
    liver function, 45, 57, 78-79, 89, 121-
        22
    other treatments, 13, 21, 22, 122,
        123
diabetes, 20, 113, 166
diet
    as detoxifying, 66
    fiber, 46, 51-52, 55, 67, 131
    fresh vs. processed, 10, 53, 62
    fruits/vegetables, 51, 63, 67, 79, 137
    as immune system supporting, 63, 66,
        126
    nursing mother's diet, 127
    overeating, 53
    recommended daily, 51, 63
    variety and, 10, 12
digestion, 42-47, 62
digestive problems, 18-20, 32, 47, 55-57, 59
    in children, 126-27, 130-31
    gastroesophageal reflux disease, 52-53
    herbal teas, 23, 35, 48, 50, 55, 56,
        130, 131
    herbal vinegars, 54, 161
    hypochlorhydria, 43, 53-55
    illness and, 20, 41-42, 62, 95
    irritable bowel syndrome, 55-56
    other treatments, 5, 13, 46-48, 55-56,
        152, 161
    see also constipation; intestinal prob-
        lems
Digestive Tonic, 54, 161
diverticular disease, 47
drug/herb interactions, 22, 35, 50, 81, 82,
    92

blood thinners, 69, 81, 99, 132
cardiac medications, 111, 113
drying herbs, 10, 12, 151, 155-56

ear problems, 131, 133
Echinacea Lemon Ginger Tea™, 67, 70, 72
eczema, 55, 57
    herbal teas, 58, 89, 99
    succus, 145
edema, 82-83
emotional imbalance, 85-89, 90-92, 100
    herbal teas, 89, 92
    hydrotherapy, 25, 87
endocrine system, *see* hormonal imbalance
epilepsy, 166
essential fatty acids (EFAs), 59, 80
essential oils, 80, 103, 137, 164-66
    cautions, 25, 26, 136, 165, 166
    eucalyptus, 100, 101, 103, 166
    fennel, 137
    hydrotherapy, 24-26, 36-37, 73, 74,
        101, 103
    lavender, 24, 27, 36-37, 73-74, 126-
        27, 165-67
    peppermint, 24-26, 73, 127, 133,
        136-37, 166
    rosemary, 25-26, 73
    tables, 26, 103
    thyme, 25-26, 73, 100-101, 103, 166
    uses, 137, 167
eucalyptus vinegar, 161
exercise, 29, 55, 72, 96, 171
expectorating herbs, 103, 106
extract solvent percentages
    arnica, 146
    calendula, 151
    chamomile, 152
    chickweed, 147
    comfrey, 147, 151
    echinacea, 153
    mint, 151
    nettles, 145, 152
    plantain, 146
    propolis, 71
    St. John's wort, 145, 153

fatigue, 20, 32, 33, 41, 44, 55, 77

herbal teas, 65, 83
hydrotherapy, 25-26
fats, 53, 55, 63
fiber, 46, 51-52, 55, 67, 131
fibrocystic breast disease, 80
first aid kit, herbal, 144-47
fixed oils, 59, 127, 147, 162, 164
flu, 64, 66
    hydrotherapy, 49-50, 104-5, 128-29
    other treatments, 69, 132
fruits, 51, 63, 67, 137

gallbladder problems, 55, 83, 123
garbling, 154
gargling, 71
Garlic Vinegar, 162
gas, 20, 44, 47, 55
    herbal tea, 48
    hydrotherapy, 49-50, 128-29
glycerine, 157-58, 160
glycerites, 155, 157-58, 160
    echinacea root, 131
    Hawthorn Berry Glycerite, 112, 114,
        160
    indications, 131, 133, 160
    shelf life, 158, 160
glycosides, 157
green clay, 141
growing herbs, 149-53

harvesting herbs, 150, 151, 153, 154-55
Hawthorn Berry Glycerite, 112, 114, 160
headaches, 18, 33
    herbal teas, 22, 23, 48, 81
    hydrotherapy, 25-26, 49-50, 74, 128-
        29, 134, 135
    other treatments, 27, 123
health and well-being, 1-4, 14-15
    as dynamic, 2, 14, 171
    food and, 10, 12
    natural cycles and, 7-9, 14, 85-87
    stress symptoms and, 17-18
heart attack, 18, 110
heartburn, 18, 43, 47, 52-55
heart function, *see* cardiovascular function
hemorrhoids, 47, 143
hepatitis, 55

herbal extracts, 157-58
see also specific kinds of extracts
Herbal Steam Inhalation for Sinuses and
     Lungs, 98, 100, 101, 103, 161, 169
herbs, 4-5, 6-7, 9
     cautions, 22, 58, 89, 113
     drying, 10, 12, 151, 155-56
     freshness and potency, 9, 10, 12, 156
     growing, 149-53
     harvesting, 150, 151, 153, 154-55
     as medicine/food, 5, 9-10, 12-13,
          139-47
     natural cycles and, 6-7, 9
HIV, 20
hoarseness, 73
homeostatic mechanism, 2-4, 14-15, 41-42,
     118, 171
honey, 137
     see also specific herbal tea recipes
hormonal imbalance, 20, 45, 55, 77-79, 80-
     83
     Castor Oil Pack Treatment, 123
     herbal teas, 80-83, 89
     herbal vinegars, 82-83
     herbs vs. hormone replacement, 77-
          78, 79
Hot Footbath for Congestive Headaches, 74
Hot Vinegar Pack, 143, 162
hydrotherapy, herbal, 24-26, 36, 51, 169
     Alternating Hot and Cold Sitz Bath,
          143
     alternating hot/cold treatments, 133,
          143
     Bath and Sweat Treatment, 72, 104-5
     benefits, 72-74, 98, 104-5, 169
     Calming Herbal Baths, 25, 134, 135
     cautions, 37, 38, 49, 89
     Constitutional Hydrotherapy Treat-
          ments, 49-50, 127, 128-29,
          169
     essential oils in, 166
     Herbal Steam Inhalation for Sinuses
          and Lungs, 98, 101, 103,
          169
     Hot Footbath for Congestive
          Headaches, 74
     Invigorating Baths, 25-26

Neutral Chamomile Bath, 25, 36, 38
Oatmeal Bath, 141, 142
Sore Throat Compress, 73
10 Minutes to Revitalization, 24
Warming Sock Treatment, 36-37, 72,
     169
hydrotherapy, *see* hydrotherapy, herbal
hyperfolin, 91
hypericin, 91
hypertension, 20, 109
     herbal teas, 113, 115
     herb cautions, 89, 166
hyperthyroidism, 55
hypoadremalism, 54
hypochlorhydria, 43, 53, 54, 55
hypotension, 113
hypothyroidism, 53, 55

Immune-Boost Cough and Cold Tea, 106,
     107
Immune Supportive Soup, 69
immune system, 62, 63-70, 72
     in children, 125-26
     depressors, 18, 20, 62-63, 67
     herbal teas, 65, 70, 72, 74, 107
     hydrotherapy, 36-37, 72-74
     other treatments, 13, 69, 161, 164
Immune Tonic Tea, 33, 64, 65, 67, 72
infertility, 20
inflammation, 113
infusions, 158, 163
     see also teas, herbal
insomnia, 18, 20, 31-33
     herbal teas, 22, 23, 33-35, 82, 152
     hydrotherapy, 36-37, 38, 49-50, 72,
          128-29, 134, 135
insulin, 44
intestinal problems, 20, 47
     herbal teas, 35, 48, 81
     herb cautions, 83
     hydrotherapy, 49-50, 128-29
     other treatments, 123
     see also digestive problems
Invigorating Baths, 25-26
irritability, 33, 35, 82, 83

joint pain, 57, 59, 89, 123, 147

Kava-Ease Tea, 21, 23
kidney function, 5, 62, 121, 152
     herbal vinegars, 161
     herb cautions, 58, 89

lactation, 83
Lavender Relaxing Bath, 87
lemon, 43, 46, 55
libido, decreased, 20
ligament injuries, 147, 151
liquids, 46, 67
Liver Cleansing Tea, 33, 52, 59, 89, 121-22,
     131
liver function, 45, 57, 78-79, 88-89, 121-22
     herbs vs. pharmaceuticals, 23, 46
     treatments, 5, 89, 122, 123, 161
Lung Cleansing Tea, 33, 97
lung function, *see* respiratory function
lupus erythematosis, 55
lymph function, 151

massage, herbal, 27, 166
meditation, 171
memory, poor, 41
menopausal symptoms, 45, 77, 80, 82, 92
menstrual discomfort, 78, 80, 82-83
     herbal teas, 23, 80, 81, 83
     hydrotherapy, 49-50
     see also premenstrual syndrome (PMS)
Menstrual Relief Tea, 80, 81
menstrums, 157-58
methylxanthines, 80
mono-amine oxidase (MAO) inhibitors, 90,
     91
mouth pain, 145
mucilaginous herbs, 100, 103, 106, 158, 168
muscle pain/spasms, 21, 41, 44, 55, 81, 141
     herbal teas, 22, 23, 35, 48, 81, 89
     herb cautions, 23, 81
     hydrotherapy, 25-26, 49-50, 128-29
     other treatments, 24, 27, 28, 145

Nasturtium Vinegar, 162
natural cycles and health, 7-9, 14, 85-87
Naturopathic medicine
     health and well-being in, 1-4, 14-15
     physicians and colleges, 131, 171

western pharmaceutical approach vs., 2, 3, 77-78, 79
whole plant vs. standardized extract, 91, 156-57
nausea, 55, 78
nervous system
    parasympathetic, 31, 43, 44, 47, 126-27
    sympathetic, 18, 19-20, 31-32, 44
nervous system imbalance, 31-32
    herbal teas, 22, 48
    hydrotherapy, 38, 49-50, 128-29
    other treatments, 13, 20, 152, 164
nettle vinegar, 152
Neutral Chamomile Bath, 25, 36, 38
New Leaf Tea™, 33, 47, 119, 120
Nutritive Vinegar for Women, 82-83

Oatmeal Bath, 141, 142
oils, fixed, 59, 127, 147, 162, 164
oils, herbal, 27, 140, 141, 155, 158, 164, 165
    arnica, 27, 140, 141, 145-46, 164
    chickweed, 147
    comfrey, 164
    St. John's wort, 164
oils, volatile, 159
organ failure, 18
osteo-arthritis, 57, 59
ovarian cysts, 123

pain, 55, 73, 145
    joint, 57, 59, 89, 123, 147
    teething, 48, 49-50, 126, 128-29, 130
    see also muscle pain/spasms
pain relief, 140
    herbal teas, 48, 59, 89, 130
    hydrotherapy, 49-50, 128-29
    other treatments, 59, 123, 145, 147, 162, 164-65
peppermint vinegar, 161
pharmaceuticals, 2, 3, 62, 85
pharmaceuticals vs. herbs, 46, 53, 61, 85, 139-40, 171
    hormone replacement, 77-78, 79
    laxatives vs. fiber, 51-52
    liver function, 46

standardized extracts, 91, 156-57
    see also drug/herb interactions
photosensitivity, 22, 90, 92
plastics, 54, 62
pneumonia
    herbal teas, 97, 107
    hydrotherapy, 100, 101, 103
    other treatments, 56
poultices, 131, 141, 155, 168
    chickweed, 147
    clay, 141
    comfrey, 131, 147, 164, 168
    garlic, 131
    ginger, 131
    plantain, 146, 167, 168
    potato/mud, 141
pregnancy, 53, 80, 82-83
pregnancy, herb cautions, 22, 35, 48, 83, 89, 99, 107, 115, 120, 123
    essential oils, 26, 166
    kava kava, 1, 23
    Oregon grape, 58, 65, 89, 107
premenstrual syndrome (PMS), 45, 77, 80
    treatments, 49-50, 82-83, 89, 123
propolis extract, 71

rashes, see skin problems
Raynaud's disease, 37, 113, 115
Red Raspberry Leaf Tea, 83
Reflexology, 27
resinous herbs, 157
respiratory function, 95-96
    see also breathing therapy
respiratory problems, 18, 20, 62, 95-96, 98-99, 133
    in children, 133, 134, 135
    herbal teas, 97, 98, 99, 100, 107
    herbal vinegars, 161, 162
    hydrotherapy, 36-37, 49-50, 72, 98, 104-5, 128-29
    hydrotherapy, steam, 100, 101, 103, 161
    infections, 100-103, 106, 107
    other treatments, 56, 100, 103, 106
restlessness, 22, 33, 38

salt use, 55, 67

salves, 155, 167-68
scars, 27
seasonal affective disorder, 77
serotonin re-uptake inhibitors (SSRIs), 90, 91
Simple Clarity™ Tea, 33, 114, 115
skin problems, 18, 55, 57, 58, 141-42
    herb cautions, 81
    hydrotherapy, 141, 142, 143
    other treatments, 58, 143, 145, 146, 147
sleep, 31-32, 36, 62
    see also insomnia
Sleep Well Tea, 34, 35
Slippery Elm Gruel, 55, 56
Slippery Elm Tea, 56
smoking, see tobacco use
somatostatin, 44
Soothing Comfort Tea™, 33, 47, 48, 50
Sore Throat Compress, 73
sore throats
    hydrotherapy, 36-37, 56, 72
    other treatments, 56, 71, 161
spearmint vinegar, 161
stage fright, 23
standardized extracts, 91, 156-57
steam inhalations, 101, 103, 166, 169
strains/sprains, see muscle pain/spasms
stress, effects of, 2-4, 14, 17-20
    cardiovascular function, 18, 20, 110
    digestion, 46-47, 54, 55
    emotional balance, 87
    immune system, 18, 20, 62, 63
    respiratory function, 96
stress
    herbal teas, 21, 22, 23, 48, 65
    hydrotherapy, 24, 25-26, 49-50, 128-29, 134, 135
    other treatments, 28-29
stressors, 19, 62
stroke, 18, 110
succuses, 140, 155, 158, 167
    calendula, 140, 144-45, 151, 158, 167
    chickweed, 147
    plantain, 158, 167
sugar use, 53, 55, 62, 67, 87, 133, 137

eliminating, 117, 119, 121, 122
    substitutes, 121, 137
Super Salad Dressing, 59, 161
surgery and herbs, 11, 82, 92, 132
Sweet Heart-Ease™ Tea, 111, 113

tannins, 158
teas, green/black, 33, 80, 158
teas, herbal, 12, 13, 155, 158, 163
    Allergy Clearing Detox Tea™, 98, 99,
        100
    calendula, 151
    chamomile, 152
    Clear Skin Tea, 58
    Cup of Sunshine Tea™, 92
    Echinacea Lemon Ginger Tea™, 67,
        70, 72
    Immune-Boost Cough and Cold Tea,
        106, 107
    immune system supporting, 65, 67
    Immune Tonic Tea, 33, 64, 65, 67, 72
    indications, 20, 46, 47, 71, 151
    Kava-Ease Tea, 21, 23
    Liver Cleansing Tea, 33, 52, 59, 89,
        121-22, 131
    Lung Cleansing Tea, 33, 97
    Menstrual Relief Tea, 80, 81
    nettles, 152
    New Leaf Tea™, 33, 47, 119, 120
    Red Raspberry Leaf Tea, 83
    Simple Clarity™ Tea, 33, 114, 115
    Sleep Well Tea, 34, 35
    Slippery Elm Tea, 56
    Soothing Comfort Tea™, 33, 47, 48,
        50
    Sweet Heart-Ease™ Tea, 111, 113
    Teething and Colic Tea, 130
    Tension Release Tea™, 22
    Women's Balance Tea, 82
Teething and Colic Tea, 130
teething pain, 48, 49-50, 126, 128-29, 130
10 Minutes to Revitalization, 24
Tension Release Tea™, 22
tinctures, 140, 141, 155, 157, 159
    nettles, 140, 141, 145, 152
    propolis extract, 71
    shelf life, 157, 159

St. John's wort, 140, 141, 145
tobacco use, 53, 63, 88, 96, 98
    eliminating, 117, 119, 120

ulcers, 18, 56
urticaria, 55
uterine fibroids, 123

vaginal dryness, 82
varicose veins, 82-83, 115
vegetables, 51, 63, 67, 79
vinegars, herbal, 114, 155, 158, 160-61, 163
    cautions, 54
    dandelion vinegar, 161
    Digestive Tonic, 54, 161
    eucalyptus vinegar, 161
    Garlic Vinegar, 162
    indications, 43, 46, 55, 114
    Nasturtium Vinegar, 162
    nettle vinegar, 152
    Nutritive Vinegar for Women, 82-83
    peppermint vinegar, 161
    shelf life, 158
    spearmint vinegar, 161
    Super Salad Dressing, 59, 161
vitiligo, 55
vomiting, 78

Warming Sock Treatment, 36-37, 72, 98,
        133, 135, 169
warts, 135, 136-37
Warts Away!, 136
weakness, 65
withdrawal symptoms, 33, 119, 120, 122
Women's Balance Tea, 82
wounds, 123, 140, 144-47, 151-52

yoga, 29, 96, 171

Herb Index

alfalfa
> immune system, 63, 64
> organ function, 79
> tea, 83

althea, respiratory function, 103

arnica, 164
> bruises, 140, 145
> cautions, 140, 146
> muscle pain/spasms, 27, 141, 145

astragalus, 66
> immune system, 65, 69
> soup, 69
> tea, 65

augustifolia, respiratory function, 103

avena, adrenal system, 79

bitter orange, sugar substitute, 137

black cobosh, hormonal balance, 79

borage, 12, 158
> joint health, 59

burdock, 12, 58, 158
> cautions, 58
> immune system, 65, 66, 69
> liver function, 79, 88, 89
> skin, 58
> soup, 69
> teas, 58, 65, 89

calendula (*Calendula officinalis*), 151, 158, 167
> emotional balance, 91, 92
> lymph function, 151
> respiratory function, 103
> wounds/burns, 140, 144-45, 151
> tea, 92

cardamom, 159
> respiratory function, 107
> tea, 107

castor bean (*Oleum ricini*), 164
> cautions, 123
> detoxification, 122, 123
> digestion, 127
> immune system, 164
> nervous system, 164
> oil packs, 122, 123, 136
> pain relief, 164, 165

skin, 137

catnip, 158, 159
> cautions, 120
> digestion, 127, 131
> tea, 119, 120
> withdrawal symptoms, 119, 120

cayenne pepper, 12, 157
> cardiovascular function, 110, 111
> immune system, 69
> soup, 69

chamomile (*Matricaria recutita, M. chamomilla*), 152
> cautions, 48, 120, 134
> digestion, 47, 48, 50, 55, 127, 130, 152
> hydrotherapy, 38, 49-50, 100-103, 134, 135, 143
> insomnia, 34, 38, 134, 152
> nervous complaints, 152
> respiratory function, 103
> skin, 143
> teas, 48, 119, 120, 130
> teething pain, 130
> withdrawal symptoms, 119, 120

chickweed (*Stellaria media*), 13
> bites, 147
> immune system, 63, 65
> organ function, 79
> skin, 146-47

cinnamon, 158, 159
> digestion, 47, 48
> gruel, 56
> respiratory function, 107
> teas, 21, 23, 58, 81, 107

cleavers
> immune system, 65
> organ function, 79

comfrey (*Symphytum officinale*), 150-51, 158, 164, 168
> bone fractures, 147, 151
> cautions, 147, 151
> ear infections, 131
> joint pain, 147
> ligaments, 147

poultice, 147, 164
> respiratory function, 103
> wounds/bruises, 147, 151

cramp bark, 157
> hormonal balance, 80, 81
> tea, 81

dandelion, 6-7, 12, 154-55, 158
> cautions, 83
> digestion, 5, 46, 52, 54, 161
> hormonal balance, 82-83
> immune system, 63, 64, 65, 161
> kidney function, 5, 161
> liver function, 5, 79, 88, 89, 161
> organ function, 79
> skin, 137
> teas, 13, 65, 82, 83, 89
> vinegars, 54, 82-83

echinacea (*Echinacea purpurea, E. augustifolia*), 153
> cautions, 70
> ear infections, 131, 133
> immune system, 13, 70, 71
> respiratory function, 103, 107, 133
> teas, 70, 107

eucalyptus, 158, 159, 166
> hydrotherapy, 100-103, 161
> respiratory function, 103, 161

evening primrose, fibrocystic breast disease, 80

eyebright
> respiratory function, 99, 133
> tea, 99

fennel, 21, 80, 159
> digestion, 47, 48, 55, 127, 131
> emotional balance, 89
> hormonal balance, 81
> immune system, 69
> muscle spasms, 21
> respiratory function, 89, 133
> soup, 69
> sugar substitute, 137
> teas, 21, 23, 33, 81, 89, 97

fenugreek
  cautions, 97
  digestion, 127
  respiratory function, 97
  tea, 97
flax, 59, 162
fox glove (*Digitalis*)
  cardiovascular function, 115
  cautions, 115
garlic, 12
  cardiovascular function, 110, 111
  cautions, 69, 132
  cough syrup, 132
  ear infections, 131
  immune system, 66, 67, 69
  respiratory function, 103, 106, 133, 162
  skin, 137
  soup, 69
  vinegars, 162
gentian, 158
  digestion, 54
  vinegar, 54
ginger, 157
  cardiovascular function, 110
  digestion, 47, 48, 127
  ear infections, 131
  emotional balance, 92
  hydrotherapy, 104-5
  immune system, 69, 70
  respiratory function, 97, 103, 104-5, 107, 133
  soup, 69
  teas, 21, 23, 58, 70, 92, 97, 107
ginkgo biloba, 13, 157
  cardiovascular function, 110, 111, 114, 115
  cautions, 92, 115
  emotional balance, 92
  teas, 92, 114, 115
ginseng, 33-34, 157
  adrenal system, 79
  cautions, 34
  nervous system, 33
goldenseal, 158
  immune system, 64
gotu kola, 157
  adrenal system, 79, 114
  cardiovascular function, 114, 115
  cautions, 115

nervous system, 33
  tea, 33, 114, 115
hawthorn, 111, 112, 157
  cardiovascular function, 110, 111, 112, 113, 114
  glycerite, 112, 114, 160
  tea, 13, 113
hellebore (veatrum)
  cardiovascular function, 115
  cautions, 115
hops, 158
  tea, 119, 120
  withdrawal symptoms, 119, 120
kava kava, 157
  cautions, 23, 81
  hormonal balance, 80, 81
  muscle relaxant, 21
  teas, 21, 23, 81
larix, ear infections, 131
lavender, 24, 159, 165, 166, 167
  cardiovascular function, 115
  cautions, 48, 115
  digestion, 47, 48, 50, 127, 130
  headache, 27
  hydrotherapy, 24, 36-37, 49-50, 73-74, 87, 134-35
  immune system, 73, 74
  insomnia, 134
  muscle tension, 24
  teas, 33, 48, 114, 115, 130
  teething pain, 126, 130
lemon balm (*Melissa officinalis*), 114, 150, 151, 159
  cardiovascular function, 110, 114, 115
  cautions, 53, 115
  digestion, 48, 50, 130
  hydrotherapy, 49-50, 134, 135
  insomnia, 134
  teas, 48, 114, 115, 130
  teething pain, 130
lemon grass
  emotional balance, 92
  immune system, 70
  teas, 70, 92
lemon verbena, tea, 22
licorice, 157
  adrenal system, 79
  cautions, 89
  digestion, 55

immune system, 65
  nervous system, 33
  respiratory function, 97, 99, 100, 103, 133
  teas, 21, 23, 33, 65, 81, 89, 97, 99
lily of the valley
  cardiovascular function, 115
  cautions, 115
milk thistle, tea, 89
motherwort, 114, 158
  cardiovascular function, 110, 111, 114
  hormonal balance, 82
  tea, 82
mullein
  ear infections, 131
  respiratory function, 103, 133
nasturtium
  respiratory function, 162
  vinegar, 162
nettles (*Urica urens*), 12, 150, 152, 155
  allergies, 145, 152
  burns, 140, 145, 152
  cautions, 99
  immune system, 63
  kidney function, 152
  organ function, 79
  respiratory function, 99, 133
  skin, 145
  teas, 83, 99
oats, 158
  cough syrup, 132
  digestion, 47, 48, 50
  headache, 50
  hydrotherapy, 49-50, 141, 142
  muscle tension/pain, 50
  nervous system, 33
  skin, 141, 142
  withdrawal symptoms, 119, 120
  teas, 33, 48, 119, 120onion, 12
  immune system, 66, 67, 69
  respiratory function, 103, 106
  soup, 69
onion, 12
  cough syrup, 32
  immune system, 66, 67, 69
  respiratory function, 103, 106
oregano
  immune system, 69
  soup, 69

Oregon grape (*Mahonia nervosa*, berberis), 158
    cautions, 58, 65, 89, 107
    digestion, 52
    emotional balance, 89
    immune system, 64, 65
    respiratory function, 103
    skin, 58
    teas, 58, 65, 89
osha
    respiratory function, 97, 103, 133
    tea, 107
parsley
    immune system, 69
    soup, 69
passion flower
    cautions, 35
    teas, 22, 35
peppermint (*Mentha piperita*), 150, 151, 158, 159, 166
    cautions, 26, 53, 120, 136
    digestion, 47, 48, 55, 127, 161
    ear aches, 133
    fatigue, 26
    hormonal balance, 82
    hydrotherapy, 24, 25-26, 73
    immune system, 73
    muscle pain/tension, 26
    pack, 136
    respiratory function, 103, 133
    skin, 136
    sugar substitute, 137
    teas, 82, 119, 120
    withdrawal symptoms, 119, 120
plantain, 158, 167, 168
    skin, 146
    wounds/burns, 146
red clover
    cautions, 99
    emotional balance, 92
    hormonal balance, 79
    liver function, 79
    respiratory function, 99, 103, 133
    teas, 92, 99
red raspberry leaf
    cautions, 83
    hormonal balance, 82-83
    immune system, 65
    tea, 83
    vinegar, 82-83

rose, 13, 112, 157
    hydrotherapy, 134, 135
    insomnia, 134
    respiratory function, 99, 100
    tea, 99
rosemary, 159
    cautions, 26
    fatigue, 26
    headache, 26
    hydrotherapy, 25-26, 73
    immune system, 69, 73
    muscle pain/tension, 26
    soup, 69
saw palmetto, hormonal balance, 79
senna
    cautions, 52
    digestion, 52
skullcap, 158
    digestion, 46, 54, 130
    teas, 22, 35, 119, 120, 130
    teething pain, 130
    vinegar, 54
    withdrawal symptoms, 119, 120
slippery elm bark, 158
    cautions, 56
    digestion, 55
    gruel, 56
    respiratory function, 103
    tea, 56
spearmint (*Mentha spicata*), 150, 151, 159
    cautions, 53
    digestion, 161
stevia
    sugar substitute, 121
    teas, 48, 70, 113, 114, 115
St. John's wort (hypericin), 90-91, 112, 153-54, 157, 164
    cautions, 22, 82, 90, 92
    detoxification, 22
    emotional balance, 13, 22, 85, 90, 91-92
    hormonal balance, 82
    liver function, 79, 88
    muscle strains/spasms, 145
    pain relief, 140, 141, 145
    skin, 145
    teas, 22, 82, 92
    wounds/burns/bruises, 140, 145
thyme, 159, 166
    cautions, 26, 50, 103
    emotional balance, 26

    fatigue, 26
    headache, 26
    hydrotherapy, 25-26, 49-50, 73, 100-101, 103
    immune system, 69, 73
    muscle pain, 26
    respiratory function, 50, 103
    soup, 69
valerian, 34
    cautions, 35, 50
    digestion, 50
    hydrotherapy, 49-50
    insomnia, 35, 50
    muscle pain/spasm, 50
    respiratory function, 103
    tea, 35
vitex berry, 157
    hormonal balance, 79, 82
    tea, 82
wild cherry bark, 158
    cautions, 107
    respiratory function, 103, 107
    tea, 107
wild yam, hormonal balance, 79
witch hazel
    hemorrhoids, 143
    hydrotherapy, 143
yellow dock
    cautions, 58
    digestion, 52
    skin, 58
    teas, 58, 89
yohimbe, hormonal balance, 79